HEALTH, WELLBEING, COMPETENCE AND AGING

ANNALS OF TRADITIONAL CHINESE MEDICINE

Series Editors: Ping-Chung Leung
(The Chinese University of Hong Kong, Hong Kong)
Charlie Changli Xue
(RMIT University, Australia)

Published

Volume 1 Chinese Medicine — Modern Practice
Edited by Ping-Chung Leung & Charlie Changli Xue
ISBN: 978-981-256-018-6
Publication date: February 2005 252 pp.

Volume 2 Current Review of Chinese Medicine: Quality Control of Herbs and Herbal Material
Edited by Ping-Chung Leung, Harry Fong & Charlie Changli Xue
ISBN: 978-981-256-707-9
Publication date: May 2006 308 pp.

Volume 3 Alternative Treatment for Cancer
Edited by Ping-Chung Leung & Harry Fong
ISBN: 978-981-270-929-5
Publication date: November 2007 384 pp.

Volume 4 Healthy Aging
Edited by Ping-Chung Leung
ISBN: 978-981-431-771-9
Publication date: October 2010 284 pp.

Volume 5 Evidence-Based Acupuncture
Edited by Tang-Yi Liu & Ping-Chung Leung
ISBN: 978-981-432-417-5
Publication date: January 2013 Approx: 204 pp.

Annals of Traditional Chinese Medicine – Vol. 6

HEALTH, WELLBEING, COMPETENCE AND AGING

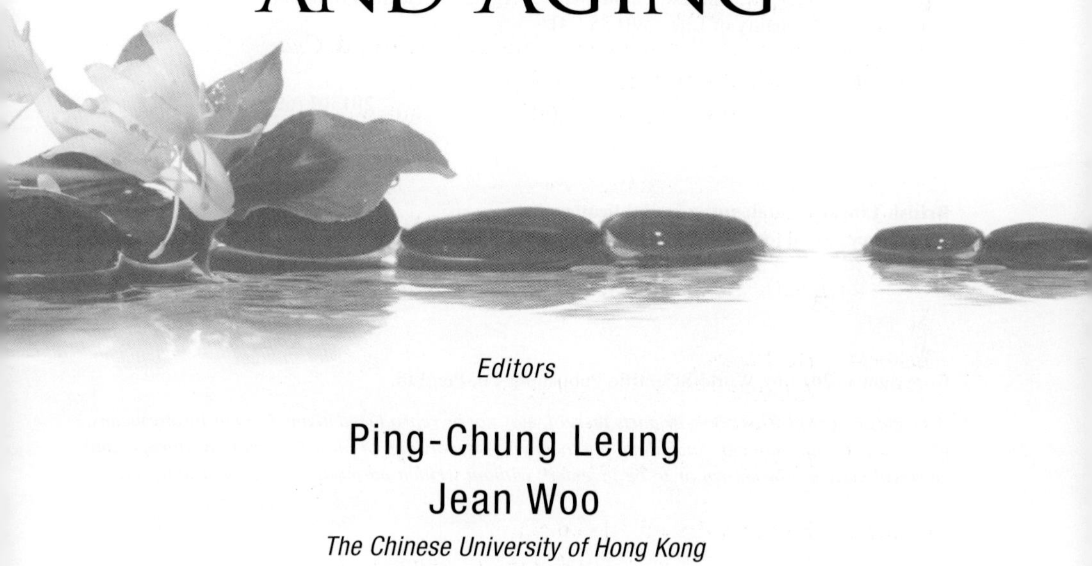

Editors

Ping-Chung Leung
Jean Woo
The Chinese University of Hong Kong

Walter Kofler
Medical University of Innsbruck and President of International Academy of Science H&E, Austria

World Scientific

NEW JERSEY • LONDON • SINGAPORE • BEIJING • SHANGHAI • HONG KONG • TAIPEI • CHENNAI

Published by

World Scientific Publishing Co. Pte. Ltd.

5 Toh Tuck Link, Singapore 596224

USA office: 27 Warren Street, Suite 401-402, Hackensack, NJ 07601

UK office: 57 Shelton Street, Covent Garden, London WC2H 9HE

Library of Congress Cataloging-in-Publication Data

Health, wellbeing, competence, and aging / edited by Ping-Chung Leung.
p. ; cm. -- (Annals of traditional Chinese medicine ; vol. 6)
Includes bibliographical references and index.
ISBN 978-9814425667 (hardcover : alk. paper)
I. Leung, Ping-Chung, 1941– editor of compilation. II. Series: Annals of traditional Chinese medicine ; v. 6.
[DNLM: 1. Medicine, Chinese Traditional. 2. Aging. 3. Health Promotion. 4. Mental Competency. 5. Quality of Life. WB 55.C4]
RA776.75
613.2--dc23

2013017693

British Library Cataloguing-in-Publication Data

A catalogue record for this book is available from the British Library.

Typeset by Stallion Press
Email: enquiries@stallionpress.com

Printed in Singapore by Mainland Press Pte Ltd.

Contents

Contributors

Kazuhiko Atsumi
The University of Tokyo
1-6-2 Mukogaoka, Bunkyo-ku
Tokyo, 113-0023, Japan

Lukas Bittner
Institute of Analytical Chemistry and Radiochemistry
CCB-Center for Chemistry and Biomedicine
Leopold-Franzens University
Innrain 80-82, 6020 Innsbruck, Austria

Agnes Suiyin Chan
Department of Psychology
The Chinese University of Hong Kong
Shatin, NT, Hong Kong

Chetwyn C. H. Chan
Laboratory of Neuropsychology
The University of Hong Kong, Hong Kong

Wai Man Chan
Rm 3502 Hopewell Centre
183 Queen's Rd East, Wanchai, Hong Kong

Leonid P. Churilov
198332 St. Petersburg
Leninskiy Prosp. Bld. 100-2, ap. 662 Russia

Christa Erhart
A-5020 Saalachstr 96, Austria

Peter Erhart
A-5020 Saalachstr 96, Austria

Dr. Ernest HM
Tai Po Hospital, Shatin, NT, Hong Kong

Nerissa S. P. Ho
Laboratory of Neuropsychology
The University of Hong Kong, Hong Kong

Christian Huck
Institute of Analytical Chemistry and Radiochemistry
CCB-Center for Chemistry and Biomedicine
Leopold-Franzens University
Innrain 80-82, 6020 Innsbruck, Austria

Walter Kofler
International Academy of Science–Health and Ecology
Meinhardstraße 10 A, 6020 Innsbruck, Austria

Chack-Fan Lee
Laboratory of Neuropsychology
The University of Hong Kong, Hong Kong

Tatia M. C. Lee
Laboratory of Neuropsychology
The University of Hong Kong, Hong Kong

Susanne Schinagl
A-5020 Saalachstr 96, Austria

David Schnaiter
Section Social Medicine, Medical University of Innsbruck
Sonnenburg Strasse 16, A-6020 Innsbruck, Austria

Stefan Schönbichler
Institute of Analytical Chemistry and Radiochemistry
CCB-Center for Chemistry and Biomedicine
Leopold-Franzens University
Innrain 80-82, 6020 Innsbruck, Austria

Kwok-Fai So
Laboratory of Neuropsychology
The University of Hong Kong, Hong Kong

Yury I. Stroev
198332 St. Petersburg
Leninskiy Prosp. Bld. 100-2, ap. 662 Russia

Sophia Laiman Sze
Department of Psychology
The Chinese University of Hong Kong
Shatin, NT, Hong Kong

Jean Woo
Division of Geriatrics, Department of Medicine and Therapeutics
The Chinese University of Hong Kong
Shatin, NT, Hong Kong

Jing Yin
Laboratory of Neuropsychology
The University of Hong Kong, Hong Kong

Ruby Yu
Division of Geriatrics, Department of Medicine and Therapeutics
The Chinese University of Hong Kong
Shatin, NT, Hong Kong

Preface to Series

Does Traditional Chinese Medicine Work?

History should be acknowledged and respected. Despite this, the historical value of Chinese medicine in China and some parts of Asia should not be used as the only important evidence of efficacy.

While clinical science has followed closely the principles of deductive research in science and developed its methodology of wide acceptance, there is a natural demand from both users and service providers that the same methodology be applied to the traditional art of healing. There should be only one scale for the measurement of efficacy. Thus, evidence-based medicine, which apparently is the only acceptable form of treatment, would also claim its sovereignty in Chinese medicine.

In spite of influential proponents and diligent practitioners, efforts relating to the application of evidence-based medicine methodology to Chinese medicine research have been slow and unimpressive. This should not come as a surprise. Evidence-based medicine requires the knowledge of the exact chemistry of the drug used, the exact physical or chemical activities involved and above all, the biological responses in the recipient. All these are not known. Working back from the black box of old historical records of efficacy requires huge resources and time, if at all possible. Insistence on this approach would result in either unending frustrations or utter desperation.

Parallel with the modern attempts, respectable Chinese medicine practitioners have unendingly and relentlessly cried out their objection to the evidence-based approach. They insisted that all the evidences were already there from the Classical Records. Forcing the classical applications through a rigid modern framework of scrutiny is artificially coating Chinese medicine with a scientific clothing that does not fit.

Thus, the modern proponents are facing an impasse when they rely totally on modern scientific concepts. The traditional converts are persisting to push their pilgrims of defense. Where do we stand so as to achieve the best results of harmonisation?

There must be a compromise somewhere. Classic evidences can be transformed into a universal language to be fairly evaluated and to be decided whether suitable for further research, using the deductive methodology or an innovative one after intelligent modifications.

There is a need for a platform on which a direction can be developed in the attempt to modernise the traditional art and science of healing, while remaining free and objective to utilise the decaying wisdom without prejudice.

With the growing demand for complementary/alternative medicine from the global public and a parallel interest from the service providers, there is an urgent need for the provision of valuable information in this area.

The Annals of Chinese Medicine is a timely serial publication responding to this need. It will be providing authoritative and current information about Chinese medicine in the areas of clinical trials, biological activities of herbs, education, research and quality control requirements. Contributors are invited to send in their reports and reviews to ensure quality and value. Clinicians and scientists who are willing to submit their valuable observations, resulting from their painstaking researches are welcome to send in their manuscripts. *The Annals of Chinese Medicine* has the objective of providing a lasting platform for all who concentrate their efforts on the modernization of Chinese medicine.

Professor Ping-Chung Leung
Institute of Chinese Medicine
The Chinese University of Hong Kong

Preface to Volume 6

Volume 6 of the *Annals of Traditional Chinese Medicine* is titled "Health, Wellbeing, Competence and Aging".

Our readers may realize that Volume 5 in this series is titled "Healthy Aging", hence an alternative to Volume 6's title would have been "Healthy Aging II". After lengthy discussions with various contributors, we finally agreed on its present title, as the elderly not only highly regard health but also wellbeing and competence in order to live happily and independently.

In October 2010, a Special International Conference dedicated to Health and Aging was held in Hong Kong. The Conference was jointly organized by the Eurasia-Pacific Uninet, an Austria-based International Network which aims to link up European and Asian Cultures, and "Multifacetal aspects of aging and age-related diseases" has been identified as a major theme since 2008. The title chosen for the conference was "Health, Wellbeing, Competence and Aging". This book is a compilation of the more important contributions from that conference. It is therefore appropriate for me to quote Prof. Dr. Brigitte Winklehner's message given at the conference:

> "The topic selected is Health, Wellbeing, Competence and Aging. We will show what new concepts of Public Health understanding can contribute to keep people healthier for a longer lifespan, assuring and maintaining the quality of life and the wellbeing of elderly humans and to put into consideration the possible ways of living arrangements — either in intergenerational co-residence, living alone or in nursing homes — in Asian and Western countries and cultures from an inter- and transcultural perspective."

Subsequently, Prof. Walter Kofler from the University of Innsbruck gave a learned account on the "Plurality of cultures and wisdom as a resource for health and competence". I quote him as follows:

> "Fundamental change in the world around us is taking place with increasing relevance to the current and further generations — but with alarming differences in the public awareness. Nearly everybody rates environmental and climate change as relevant danger to health, wellbeing and quality of life for him/herself, the family and as a local and global problem because of their direct and indirect effects. Therefore governments and networks of powerful NGOs all over the world cooperate within and for international agreements (e.g. Kyoto Protocol) in order to create solutions on individual, familial, local and global levels. But why is such an awareness missing from the basic current demographic shift which will take place during the next 40 years? Its direct and indirect consequences on health, quality of life and wellbeing are not less relevant as the ecological changes. For 2050 an increase of the world wide population from about seven billion up to about nine billion people is predicted, with an extreme increase of senior citizens up to about two billion. Curative health care is for both types of changes — the environmental one as well as the demographic one — a necessary answer — but this answer alone would be totally insufficient. This demonstrates dementia, the most relevant epidemic, which is predicted for the coming decades. The costs for the informal care are a multiple of the costs for traditional health care. But these financial costs are not the most relevant aspect. Dementia dominates not only the daily life and wellbeing of the ill person but can also affect the life of the associated family members by two to three times."

We should understand aging not just as a social danger but also as a challenge. The predominant part of the process of growing old is healthy. It is within our means to adjust our behavior and value systems early enough to a more appropriate mindset towards aging; in this context we can learn a lot from other cultures.

We have to understand the plurality of cultures, knowledge and ways of life as resources to learn from each other. Such a position can be a basis for a new type of solidarity as a tool for a more appropriate means of coping with the challenges of the future. Therefore we plan, in cooperation with the World Aging Forum, to create bulletins with reference to these aspects. A bulletin is a report of experts about the health situation of a high standing person; our bulletins should deal with the situation of mankind with respect to lifelong health and with respect to socio-cultural plurality. We will start with the Hong Kong Bulletin for Lifelong Health: Healthy and Competent Aging. This bulletin should be created on the basis of the results of this conference. All representatives are invited to give us recommendations what could be offered by their cultural experiences to deal more appropriately with aging.

Such a transcultural discussion should be started with a presentation of the scientific self-understanding, which is given in the cultural regions of the key discussion partners: health and wellbeing in general, and in the special context of senior citizens, bodily, psychic, social, cultural, ecological, political, etc. influences on and its interactions with a comprehensive ("holistic") response. We have to expect differences in the handling of such interactions. Therefore, it is necessary to introduce both the western and eastern scientific self-understanding, and to link the different responsible aspects for a more appropriate understanding of the very complex interactions, which finds its visible expression in the special status of an individual or in the different aspects of health within a community or a society.

Under the broad framework suggested by the two Austrian Professors, we have organized the manuscripts in an order that would probably help our readers to follow the transcultural perspectives of Health, Wellbeing, Competence and Aging.

Professor Ping-Chung Leung
Institute of Chinese Medicine
The Chinese University of Hong Kong

Chapter 1

Chinese Medicine has a Lot to Offer

Ping-Chung Leung

Abstract

Aging is a normal physiological process. The factors affecting aging are extremely complex, involving innate genetic, pathological, social-psychological and environmental factors.

Chinese Medicine takes a philosophical view on health that is considered a harmonious balanced state of physiological functions. Maintaining this balance is an effective way of preventing diseases. The balance is favorably maintained through a careful choice of dietary components and a smart practice of exercises which go beyond the usual concept of training muscles and physical abilities. Now that life expectancy is ever increasing, the awareness of wellness and disease prevention has gained universal interests. Apparently, the popular concerns of health promotion viz. cardiovascular, anti-aging, bone health, etc. can be satisfied through a Chinese way of non-aerobic exercises and practical selection of health supplements.

Keywords: Chinese Medicine; Herbs; Prevention; Exercises; Health Supplements.

Knowledge about Chinese Medicine has been misleading. In Europe and America, Chinese Medicine might mean acupuncture and a collection of proprietary botanical drugs manufactured from medicinal herbs. For the Koreans, Chinese Medicine has been adopted in ancient Korea and developed with refinement into "Oriental Medicine". For the Japanese, Chinese Medicine was the mainline clinical tool before and during the Edo period. Since then Kampo Medicine based on Chinese Medicine has replaced it. Of course a traditional practice could take different forms of development but its cultural roots would ever remain. Given its very long history of record keeping, extending from 3000 years ago, and with numerous occasions of integration with clinical streams outside China during the many imperial efforts of trade expansion along the "Silk route" in the different dynasties, Chinese Medicine very much represents an amalgamation of clinical wisdom in Central China, as well as those collected from India, Persia and around the Mediterranean. Among the different systems of Traditional Medicine, therefore, Chinese Medicine is the broadest and most integrative. The rich historical background and the tremendous collection of clinical wisdom and facts must have perpetuated the popularity and everlasting value of Chinese Medicine (Bensky and Gamble, 1993).

Yet, surprisingly, today, when one takes a careful check at the practice within the most respectable establishment of Chinese Medicine, viz. any "Chinese Medicine Hospital" in China, one's impression would be that of confusion.

Since the establishment of these "Chinese Medicine Hospitals" in China around the 1950s, they have been providing Chinese Medicine services. Historically traditional Chinese Medicine services were not given in hospital settings. In reality the so-called "Chinese Medicine Hospitals" of today are all mixed hospitals giving both Western and Chinese Medicine services. The very busy outpatient clinics offer mostly Chinese Medicine services like acupuncture and herbal treatment. Once admitted into the wards, the treatment would be mainly modern medicine because of the need for acute management and life-saving procedures. Chinese Medicine practitioners are making their greatest contributions in pain control, cancer adjuvant therapy, allergic conditions, aging and other odd disease pathologies. Their services can be focused mostly in those areas, however they do not want to limit their services. The result is that they need to make use of modern medicine to maintain a comprehensive claim.

The reason behind the bending of traditional practice towards the modern, technology-based approach is also related to financial balance. To sustain a modern hospital, a lot of resources are required. Now that China requires every hospital to be financially independent, relying only on manual therapy, acupuncture and/or herbal remedy would not be sufficient to make ends meet, much less profit. The only means for the Chinese Medicine Hospitals to survive, therefore, is to offer profitable services like modern investigations, surgical interventions, expensive pharmaceuticals, etc.

Chinese Medicine is a pride to all Chinese people because of its obvious link to Chinese culture and philosophy. The pride expands as people outside China are looking up to unique practices like acupuncture, and more and more people are using self-prescribed herbal supplements although some of which might not have originated from Chinese Medicine at all.

Chinese Medicine would stay as a national pride in China, with or without government protection. On the service side, it is already clear that it has a lot to offer in aging and chronic problems, pain control, neurological deficits and other situations when modern treatment fails. Degeneration is an inevitable physiological process associated with aging. Degeneration has the general aspect where tissues and organs run a gradual degradation (Stewart *et al.*, 1989; Kaptchuk and Eisenberry, 1988). Degeneration commonly affects a special functional component of normal physiological activity like the cardiovascular function, musculoskeletal integrity, and mental ability. Chinese Medicine has the traditional claim of maintaining an internal harmony, which refers to a general maintenance of physiological balance. It is also well-known that special choices of herbal combinations have been used traditionally for cardiovascular health, muscle and joint strength, and mental well-being. In the current context, therefore, Chinese Medicine has a lot to offer in those areas.

Oriental societies have a long history of promoting health through the prevention of diseases, which are not short of special terms and connotations. Thus for Traditional Chinese Medicine (TCM), "treating diseases before their onset" does not refer to what we understand by the Public Health Standards of disease prevention, but points to a more personalized pursuit of good health before an individual is disease-struck. Under this category of health practice, living and eating habits, lifestyles and special supplements, are all considered. In fact TCM practitioners consider food to be a form of medicine, and the Indian Ayurvedic practitioners are equally conscious about lifestyle and diet (Su, 1992; Dahanuakr and Thatte, 1996).

"Treating diseases before their onset" requires the individual to be aware of his/her current state of health: whether there is objective or subjective feeling of deficiencies or symptoms, which could then be specifically watched and contained using non-therapeutic means. Such feeling of health risk might refer to frailty, cardiovascular deficiency, joint and bone deterioration, over-weight or loss of mental acuity, etc. (Jiang, 2002).

1.1 Food as Medicine

Traditional Chinese Medicine has long history of categorizing varieties of food as medicine-like items which offer specific benefits to different health demands. Classically such food categories are used for the supplement of various deficiencies within "*qi*", "*yin*" and "*yang*", which represent heart-felt philosophical expressions rather than specific symptoms. With modern knowledge, the philosophical expressions could be translated into modern language describing different symptomatologies related to physiological systems and structural pathologies.

To give some common examples, see Table 1.1, which lists the herbal items advocated for general and unique health needs. The listed herbal items include commonplace vegetables used in day-to-day meals, as well

Table 1.1. List of Chinese medicinal herbs used as food and health supplements.

Function	Herbal items
General support	*Radix Ginseng*
	Radix Codonopsis
	Rhizoma Dioscoreae
	Semen Nelumbinis
	Rhizoma Polygonati Odorati
	Bulbus Lilii
	Semen Coicis
	Semen Sesami Nigrum
	Fructus Crataegi
	Adenophora Stricta
Supplementing hemopoiesis	*Angelica sinensis*
	Radix Polygoni Multiflori
	Fructus Lycii
Supplementing *yin*	*Fructus Ligustri Lucidi*
	Rhizoma Polygonati Odorati
	Radix Astragalus
	Cordyceps
Supplementing *yang*	*Cortex Eucommiae*
	Cornu Cervi Pantotrichum
	Herba Epimedii

as rarer herbal items better known in the traditional medicine circle (Liang and Liang, 2006).

These herbs are known to have general supportive effects. Some are popular among the male or female. The most accepted utilizations include the supplement of physiological imbalance, described as *yin* and *yang* excess or deficiency (Guan *et al.*, 2008).

Outside Asia, medicinal herbs might be better known as ingredients for cooking rather than being considered as food. Some herbs are well known to have special therapeutic effects (John, 1974). Table 1.2 contains a list of some common examples.

Table 1.2. Therapeutic effects of some common foods.

Indication	Food	Indication	Food
Anemia	Alfalfa	Blood pressure	Onion
	Artichoke		Garlic
	Chive		Anise
Allergy	Papaya		Hawthorn
	Perilla	Bruises	Aloe
Appetite	Anise		Celery
	Cranberry		Pine-apple
	Black pepper	Colds	Ginger
	Celery		Ginseng
	Mint		Licorice
Cardiovascular health	Garlic	Constipation	Asparagus
	Hawthorn		Flax
	Onion		Plum
	Olive	Diabetes	Chicory
Joint pain	Horseradish		Dandelion
	Blackcurrant		Artichoke
Asthma	Peony	Diarrhea	Sage
	Parsley		Basil
	Almond		Cinnamon fern
Backpain	Black cohosh	Toothache	Clove
	Oat		Hops
	Mustard		

1.2 Health Claims and Efforts to Regulate Claims

The quest for better health and longevity is well appreciated by the commercial world. The popular traditional practice of cooking and the use of medicinal herbs are modified today as user-friendly health supplements in the convenient forms of tablets, capsules and drinks. Supermarkets are displaying shelf after shelf of health supplements with special health claims, which vary from sheer advertising to traditional beliefs with or without modern justifications. Claims rely on a number of channels: from literature search on health use, laboratory results, animal observations and simple user experiences, all of which possess only low levels of evidence (Bellisle *et al.*, 1998).

The flourishing business of health supplements has naturally invited the attention of regulators who need to control misleading advertising and to protect the users. We should look at the recommendations established in Europe, the US and China.

1.2.1 *European Union*

Since 2001, Health Authority in the European Union started to work on the recommendations to be given for the justification of health claims for health supplements. Large powerful working committees were established to be responsible, and after five years, a proper document was created (COM, 2003).

Seven specific areas were identified, viz. cardiovascular, bone health, physical fitness, body weight regulation, cancer prevention, mental performance and gastrointestinal health, for special scrutiny. With regard to the procedures required for the assessment of health claims (PASSCLAIM), three major foci are chosen: (1) the essential components of the food or health supplement itself, (2) the biological effects of the food or health supplements as observed in the laboratory, and (3) the eventual reduction of disease risks.

It is clear that foci (1) and (2) involve literature search and laboratory work which are easy to achieve, but to prove reduction of disease risk might need proper clinical trials of long durations and high costs. The European Authority acknowledged the difficulty and suggested compromising considerations of small, low level human trials with accumulative data (Aggett *et al.*, 2005).

1.2.2 *United States*

In the United States, there is yet no generally accepted recommendation for the registration of health food and health supplements. In 2003, the American Association of Clinical Endocrinologists (AACE) worked out a set of medical guidelines for the clinical use of dietary supplements and neutraceuticals (AACE, 2003). The guidelines were compiled according to expert opinions which actually followed closely practices of clinical investigations and new drug discovery. The evaluation of the trustworthiness of health supplements was based on three levels of observations. Level 3 refers to all available information related to the clinical benefits including simple case reports. Level 2 refers to simple clinical trials, whether properly or not properly organized. The highest level of Level 1 refers to randomized control trials and meta-analysis. With such understanding, one wonders whether the guidelines are in fact full strict regulations as are required in drug evaluations (Goodman, 2002).

AACE gave a number of examples which are popular non-descriptive supplements claiming specific effects like cholesterol control, glucose control, menopausal well-being, anti-depression, etc. With such specific indications, it is no wonder why the AACE is taking views not different from drug discovery (Engel, 1977).

1.2.3 *China*

The State Food and Drug Administration of China (SFDA) has a well defined set of regulations for the registration of health food and supplements (SFDA, 2002). Since China has a large number of food and medicinal herbs consumed as food, SFDA grouped the herbs into three categories, viz. those used as food, those used either as food or drug, and those that should not be used as food.

With this specific grouping the regulating authority would have less difficulty doing the assessment, however, the procedures required for an official registration are still cumbersome and restrictive. A lot of official reports need to be submitted, including: a detailed description of the item to be registered; additives; special requirements with special plants and animals; toxicology reports, etc. There is however, no requirement on the efficacy explanation or justification of health claims.

The strong tradition of "food therapy" in China must have influenced both users and regulators on their free attitude and trust on the value of health supplements so that as long as their use is along the traditional line, no specific requirements are imposed (Li *et al.*, 2006).

1.3 How Should Health Claims be Justified?

Health claims could be made on anything that is involved in a popular health pursuit that could be fashionable or circumstantial. Thus, slimming could be a fashionable demand leading to slimming supplements while spring-time influenza and the fear of contracting it could initiated a circumstantial pursuit for "anti-flu" supplements.

The European Union, during its establishment of the PASSCLAIM, selected specific areas of concern which were believed to be popular and important. The areas include cardiac health, musculoskeletal degeneration, bone health, frailty, obesity, Gastrointestinal comfort and cancer prevention. It is obvious that five of the selected areas are related to aging, while cancer phobia probably affects every individual.

The European Authority has taken a most practical approach to regulate the producers who are committing their business on health supplements according to popular needs.

Academics on Nutritional Studies have put a lot of emphasis on food and supplements that could be demonstrated to possess antioxidant effects. Antioxidants are assumed to be capable of clearing oxidized wastes, thus maintaining tissue viability, preserving energy, counteracting inflammation, and even preventing cancer formation (Ristow *et al.*, 2009). However, long term observations have revealed that antioxidants might prevent the health-promoting effects of physical exercises; might have little or no effects on the risks of developing common cancers and cardiovascular diseases; do not affect disease mortality; and importantly, some antioxidants might promote odd metabolic disturbances like renal stones (Taylor *et al.*, 2004). Choosing health supplements according to their laboratory evidence of some specific biological function like antioxidation, might then appear inappropriate or even risky.

When we look at the old philosophical beliefs in Traditional Chinese Medicine, we find that food is considered as a health supplement, and special food is recommended for special needs. The herbal items used either as food or health supplement are consumed to maintain an internal physiological balance, instead of inducing some specific activity. The current observations of antioxidants inducing harmful effects rather than health promotion could be examples of over-activity in normally balanced physiological states. The modern interpretation of physiological balance (or *yin-yang* harmony in Chinese Medicine Context) could be a state of immunological balance.

As food and health supplements are being assessed for their health claims, perhaps special attention could be put on their effects on immunological modulation (Kaminogawa and Nanno, 2004). The information is obtainable both in the laboratory and in clinical settings. Many herbal items have already been studied and found to possess immuno-modulating effects in either up-regulating or down-regulating fashions (Patarca, 2001; Field *et al.*, 2002). Well known examples include products of fungus origin like coriolus, maitake, cordyceps and medicinal roots like turmeric and astragalus.

These food and health supplements affect the immunological system either via an innate pathway, bolstering the phagocytic activity of white cells or activating N-K cells, or via an acquired initiation of T cell responses or antibody production (Kaminogawa and Nanno, 2004).

1.4 Self-Help Exercise to Maintain Health

I have discussed Taichi and Qi Gong in "*Healthy Aging*", Vol. 4 of the series which this book is part. I have tried to analyze the contents of different forms of self-performed exercises popular in Asia as different from the counterparts in Europe and America, which involve much more energy expenditure. If oriental exercises are mainly composed of three components, viz. stretching of muscles, tendons and integuments; controlled breathing; and meditation, stretching could be related to the proprioceptive related neuro-physiological phenomenon of "gate theory" through which pain control and well-being are achieved. Controlled breathing brings about a close correlation between the somatic and autonomic nervous systems, hence, with sustained practice, it initiates a state of extreme mental serenity that is usually achieved through meditation exercises with special training. The different forms of self-performed stretching and breathing exercises therefore serve the elderly people very well in their attempts to maintain health and longevity.

Stretching intensely mobilizes the tissues along the direction of pull; likewise, the interstitial tissues are also involved. A broad term "fascia" has been used as an anatomical description of the interstitial tissues. The recent understanding about the fascia and its related physiological importance has brought new light on a further explanation of the effects of stretching involved in the various forms of self-performed training exercises.

> "Fascia is the soft tissue component of the connective tissue system that permeates the human body. The scope of our definition of and interest in fascia extends to all fibrous connective tissues, including aponeuroses, ligaments, tendons, retinaculae, joint capsules, organ and vessel tunics, the epineurium, the meninges, the periostea, and all the endomysial and intermuscular fibers of the myofasciae (Huijing *et al.*, 2009)."

Rather than having to draw arbitrary demarcation lines between joint capsules and their intimately involved ligaments and tendons (as well as interconnected aponeuroses, retinacula and intramuscular fasciae), fascial tissues are seen as one interconnected tensional network that adapts its fiber arrangement and density according to local tensional demands.

Joint motion mechanically affects nerves. The nerve receptors have traditionally been divided into muscle or joint receptors; however, a continuum of receptor types can be seen across both tissues, defined by the types of stresses borne by the specific tissue. There are four classes of nerve receptors: muscle spindles; Golgi tendon organs and Ruffini corpuscles; lamellated or paciniform corpuscles; and free nerve endings. The first three classes are found in muscles, the latter three in the connective tissue surrounding joints.

Considering the types of receptors which are sensitive to dynamic force changes in compression (the laminated corpuscles) and tension or torsion (the spray-type endings), and whether such endings adapt slowly or rapidly to loading or have low or high thresholds, can help in the development to hypotheses regarding potential effects of therapy on the inputs to the nervous system. Motion at either the hip or the ankle results in nerve motion not only at the joint moving but also at more distant joints. Motion at the hip combined with motion at the ankle results in higher strains in the nerves at the ankle to levels that can impair blood flow, even in normal nerves (Huijing *et al.*, 2009).

There is epimuscular myofascial force transmission. Activation of the flexor pollicis longus (FPL), a muscle unique to human primates that contributes to manual dexterity by independently flexing the thumb, resulted in a load on the index finger about 5% of the force level of the thumb. This occurred without any time delay, which would be expected if the force transfer was through a viscoelastic mechanical connection between the muscles (Huijing *et al.*, 2009).

For some muscles tenotomy changes the maximally shortened length by only 1.5%, compared with a 4% decrease after muscle dissection. Within a muscle fiber, up to half of the total force generated by the muscle is transmitted to surrounding connective tissues rather than directly to the origin and insertion of the muscle fibers. Force can be transmitted to adjacent muscles that are synergistic, as well as to extramuscular tissues such as the neurovascular tract and various septa and membranes; by this extramuscular pathway, such forces can reach antagonistic muscles (Huijing *et al.*, 2009).

Cells can activate internal chemical signaling pathways, increase stress-fiber assembly and adhesive strength, and form focal adhesions in response to externally applied mechanical forces. Ordinarily this mechanism is damped to lower the sensitivity of this mechanism to normal physiologic fluctuations. However, once a large-scale change occurs in the cell shape, that cell then becomes more responsive to its immediate mechanical domain (Huijing *et al.*, 2009).

Differentiated cells contact and move within matrices whose stiffness ranges from as soft as the brain to as firm as collagen-coated glass. Among already differentiated cells, fibroblasts are the most responsive to the stiffness of the matrix, but undifferentiated stem cells are even more influenced. Mesenchymal stem cells (MSCs) are bone marrow-derived adult stem cells that can differentiate into neurons, myoblasts and osteoblasts. Depending on the force required to deform the matrix, neurogenic, myogenic, or osteogenic RNA transcriptional markers are produced if, respectively, the matrix is soft (brain-like, 1 kPa elasticity), more rigid (muscle-like, 10 kPa), or stiff (bone-like, 100 kPa). The myosin genes appear sensitive to matrix stiffness, so that as the matrix becomes stiffer, more myosin is produced, allowing the cell to generate sufficient force to accommodate an up-to-100-times difference in stiffness. Blood flow to tissues rapidly increases when muscles contract through local mechanisms (Huijing *et al.*, 2009).

Actively contracting skeletal muscle generates tensile forces that change the conformation of fibronectin fibers surrounding the arteriolar wall. Contraction of one muscle within the compartment results in a small elevation of pressure, which increase contractile efficiency of the other muscles contained within that compartment. These normal pressure changes result in cyclical changes throughout the gait cycle, which assists in venous return of blood to the heart with the calf muscles serving as a "second heart pump" (Casey and Hart, 2008; Panny *et al.*, 2009). Fascial envelopes of peripheral nerve fascicles (perineurium, which maintains the so-called blood-nerve barrier) as well as the much thicker layer surrounding whole peripheral nerves with their blood supply (epineurium). These two fascial layers are themselves innervated by "nervi nervorum", which can evoke nociception and are likely responsible for nerve trunk pain. They can also evoke neurogenic inflammation. The inflammatory response is limited to the epi- and perineurium and outlasts the axonal mechanical sensitivity by months.

Although the pain generative role of spinal disc damage is undisputed for some cases of low back pain, they do not seem to play a decisive role in the majority of cases in this very common pathology. Comparisons of lumbar spine MRI between back pain patients and normal patients reveal that many people without back pain show severe disc damage as well, and many back pain patients on the other side show significantly better discs than comparable pain-free people of the same age group (Jensen *et al.*, 1994). Inflammatory processes in the lumbar fasciae could be the main generation cause of low back pain. The low back pain group had a 25% greater perimuscular connective tissue thickness and echogenicity than the pain-free control group.

These novel findings of fascial anatomy and function have provided more information about the stretching of muscles, tendons, ligaments, and nerves. The fascial system which contains all those structures appears to be the dynamic origin of neurological, cellular and molecular activities which occur simultaneously with stretching. Those activities are apparently related to pain control, tissue repair and regeneration.

1.5 Discussion

Aging is a normal physiological process. It cannot be eliminated; it could only be slowed down. Scientists are working very hard to find out the genomic and molecular targets responsible for aging; their aim is to get rid of them after their identification. In the animal experiment platforms, scientists believe they are getting nearer and nearer to the identification of such aging-related molecular targets. Some experimental platforms have even demonstrated the possibility of removing the aging genes (Bordone and Guarente, 2005; Kaeberlein *et al.*, 1999).

While optimism is growing, one must realize that factors affecting aging must be extremely complex. Biologically, multiple targets must be responsible. The complexity is further complicated by the external environment which keeps changing all the time.

Scientists in the phytochemistry field have been working hard to identify small chemical molecules in the complicated herbal extracts found to be effective in maintaining health in the conventional enthusiasm of drug discovery. Proponents of traditional herbal formulation, on the other hand, have been working out bioactive fractionations to facilitate the justification of symptom control using those formulae or their modifications. While breakthrough successes in drug discovery is expected, and better and better proprietary preparations derived from original herbal formulae will be available, well-planned eating habits with carefully selected food items could still serve the aging population well. Enhanced merits will also be expected when careful eating is coupled with self-maintained stretching exercises with controlled breathing.

Chinese Medicine started as philosophical concerns related to health. It relies on the maintenance of an internal physiological balance which is essential for the stability of vital activities and is the best means of preventing deterioration. While aging with deteriorating health and degeneration of tissues and organs seem inevitable, the Chinese Medicine way of keeping the physiological balance through careful eating, controlled lifestyles and self-maintained exercises appears to be the most comprehensive and economic way of attaining longevity to be recommended.

References

Aggett, P.J., Antoie, J.M. and Bellisle, F., *et al.* (2005) Passclaim. Consensus on criteria. *Eur. J. Nutr.* **44**(S1), I/5–I/30.

American Association of Clinical Endocrinologists. (2003) Medical guidelines for the clinical use of dietary supplements and nutraceuticals. *Endocr. Pract.* **9**(5), 417–470.

Bellisle, F., Diplock, S.T. and Hornstra, G., *et al.* (1998) Functional food science in Europe. *Br. J. Nutr.* **80**(S1), 1–2.

Bensky, D. and Gamble, A. (1993) *Chinese Herbal Medicine: Materia Medica.* Eastland Press, Seattle, 1993, pp. 124–158.

Bordone, L. and Guarente, L. (2005) Calorie restriction, SIRT1 and metabolism: understanding longevity. *Nat. Rev. Mol. Cell. Biol.* **6**(4), 298–305.

Casey, D.P. and Hart, E.C. (2008) Cardiovascular function in humans during exercise: role of the muscle pump. *J. Physiol.* **586**(21), 5045–5046.

Commission Proposal for a Regulation of the European Parliament and of the Council on nutrition and health claims made on foods; COM (2003) 424 final COD 2003/0165 of 18 July 2003.

Dahanuakr, S. and Thatte U. (1996) *Ayurveda Unravelled.* Natural Book Trust, India.

Engel, G.L. (1977) The need for a new medical model: a challenge for biomedicine. *Science* **196**, 129–136.

Field, C.J., Johnson, I.R. and Schley, P.D. (2002) Nutrients and their role in host resistance to infection. *J. Leukoc. Biol.* **71**(1), 16–32.

Goodman, N.W. (2002) Criticizing evidence-based medicine. *Thyroid* **10**(2), 157–160.

Guan, D.Q., Huang, Y.Z. and Sun, Y.J. (2008) *Nutrient Value of Foods — Chinese: Most Consumed Common Foods in Hong Kong*. New Talents Press, Hong Kong.

Huijing, P.A., Hollander, P., Findley, T.W. and Schleip, R. (2009) *Fascia Research II: Basic Science and Implications for Conventional and Complementary Health Care.* Elsevier Urban and Fischer, Munich, Germany, pp. 2–12.

Jensen, M.C., Brant-Zawadzki, M.N., Obuchowski, N., Modic, M.T., Malkasian, D. and Ross, J.S. (1994) Magnetic resonance imaging of the lumbar spine in people without back pain. *N. Engl. J. Med.* **331**(2), 69–73.

Jiang, W. (2002) The ideas of "treating disease before its onset". *J. Nanjing Univ. Tradit. Chin. Med.* **18**, 209–210.

John, B.L. (1974) *The Herb Book*. Bantam Book, New York.

Kaeberlein, M., McVey, M. and Guarente, L. (1999) The SIR 2/3/4 complex and SIR 2 alone promote longevity in *Saccharomyces cerevisiae* by two different mechanisms. *Genes Dev.* **13**, 2570–2580.

Kaminogawa, S. and Nanno, M. (2004) Modulation of immune functions by foods. *Evid. Based Complement. Altern. Med.* **1**(3), 241–250.

Kaptchuk, T.J. and Eisenbery D.M. (1988) The persuasive appeal of alternative medicine. *Ann Intern. Med.* **129**(12)**,** 1061–1065.

Li, H.L., Wang, Y. and Tsao, W.K. (2006) Health food's development and material safety. *Food Sci.* **27**(3), 263–266.

Liang, S.M. and Liang, S.Q. (2006) *Anti-Ageing Herbs*. Natural Health Press, Hong Kong.

Panny, M., Ammer, K., Kundi, M., Katzenschlager, R. and Hirschl, M. (2009) Severity of chronic venous disorders and its relationship to the calf muscle pump. *Vasa* **38**(2), 171–176.

Patarca, R. (2001) Cytokines and chronic fatigue syndrome. *Ann. N. Y. Acad. Sci.* **933**, 185–200.

Ristow, M., Zarse, K. and Oberbach, A. *et al.* (2009) Antioxidants prevent health-promoting effects of physical exercise in humans. *Proc. Natl. Acad. Sci. USA* **106**(21), 8665–8670.

State Food and Drug Administration of China (SFDA), Ministry of Health of The People's Republic of China. (2002) Further regulation on the control of food material. *Health Legislation*, No. 51. [in Chinese]

Stewart, A.L., Greenfield, R.D. and Hays, R.D. *et al.* (1989) Functional status and well being of patients with chronic conditions. *J. Am. Med. Assoc.* **262**, 907–913.

Su, W.T. (1992) *History of Drugs*. United Medical University Press, Beijing.

Talyor, E.N., Stampfer, M.J. and Curhan, G.C. (2004) Dietary factors and the risk of incident kidney stones in men: new insights after 14 years of follow-up. *J. Am. Soc. Nephrol.* **15**(12), 3225–3232.

Chapter 2

Extended View of a Bio-Psycho-Socio-Eco-Cultural Model and the Self-Understanding of Western Medicine and New Public Health

Walter Kofler

Abstract

This contribution deals with the underestimated relevance of accepted scientific fundamentals of Western Medicine on its efficiency. These fundamentals restrict in principle the options to promote aging in competence, health and wellbeing; therefore, a scientific technique is presented to extend the given performance. This "Extended View" opens the door to additional hints which can be given by Oriental scientific offers.

Keywords: Theory of Science; Ontology; Epistemology; Monism; Real Theories; Evolution.

2.1 History

The state of knowledge is an actual spotlight on a process — only to be understood with respect to the process. This process is influenced by scientific, epistemological/ontological and socio-cultural aspects (e.g. based on religions) and their interactions.

2.1.1 *The Christian churches were responsible for ideational aspects — scientists (only) for material aspects*

The actual self-understanding of natural sciences can merely be understood with respect to historic interactions between science and the Christian churches: The churches claimed the monopoly of distinguishing between true and not true and, therefore, of all that was linked to logic thinking. The political power in the Western world supported this position up to the end of the 19th century. The first proposal which allowed extending scientific work on special aspects of the human mind was given by Descartes. He distinguished two different substances (materialistic dualism): *res cogitans* and *res extensa*. *Res cogitans* allows us to explain the logical aspect of a person, including its soul. The research on it was reserved to the clerus. *Res extensa* explains the somatic aspects, including the aspects of life and emotion and, therefore, unobservable aspects too (Descartes and Wohlers, 2005). In the 19th century, physical, chemical and somatic processes were explained with a mechanistic model and various types of consumable energy like forces and power. Life processes and emotions were explained in a similar way: *vis vitalis* is an invisible but consumable force. As soon as *vis vitalis* was consumed the living being died. In the special case of a human person the final rest of *vis vitalis* was used to exhale the "immortal soul (= *res cogitans*). This substance-dualistic position was falsified by the evolutionary theory of Darwin (Darwin, 1871, first published in 1859): *Vis vitalis* could no longer be unchangeable, if the structure is to be understood in an evolutionary based way. And there were no confirmations for the assumption that *vis vitalis* should be identical in all living beings.

But this scientific conclusive argumentation was not accepted immediately by society; even scientific societies insisted in the theological position of a creation of the world in six days as written in the nearly three thousand years old Genesis. For example the professor for anatomy and embryology Roux (chair-holder at the University of Innsbruck between 1889 and 1895) got his cathedra only after having himself obliged not to teach Darwin's theory (Schmidt, 2004).

Evolutionary theory could not explain adequately the autopoiesis of life, mind, free will, etc. Many propositions were offered in the 19th century and later to handle the dilemma between "science" and the "officially accepted" worldview. The proposal of the famous physiologist E. du Bois-Reymond (1872) is well known: He accepted in principle an invisible force to explain the ability to think as he accepted invisible forces to explain physical phenomena. He deduced from a modification of the philosophy of I. Kant: Because of the *a priori* given physiological limitations of the human nature, we do not know and will never know on a level which is comparable with our knowledge about physical forces where the invisible force to think, e.g. movement and sensation, life, free will, etc., come from, therefore it would be a waste of time and money to deal with the so-called world riddles (Du Bois-Reymond, 1882). With this publication an intense epistemological discussion was started in the westerns scientific community ("the so-called "ignorabimus-discussion"). But there was a relevant consequence for natural scientists: The position of du Bois-Reymond allowed to bridge the gap between the social need not to do research dealing with aspects of *res cogitans* and the acceptance that there should be in principle the same chain of argumentation for a sufficient explanation even for intellectual, emotional and cognitive effects. But the final reaction of the western scientists was more radical — if we are not able to deal with them, then we cannot confirm their existence. Therefore it is better to exclude all aspects which cannot be observed (including all discussions about philosophy including ontology) from natural science (positivism).

In the meantime Einstein had been able to falsify partly one of these "Ignorabimus" and today the Christian churches are no longer a limiting factor for scientific research. However, after about 1920 natural science did not systematically deal with its ontological and epistemological fundaments anymore. Therefore the scientific community accepts the explanation of physical and chemical processes with invisible forces, fields and powers, but does not accept such invisibles in biology, ethology, etc.

2.1.2 *Limitations of scientific explanations based on historic definitions and ontologies*

This historic excursion is not only relevant for the actual understanding of the self-understanding of western medicine, but in part highlights some of the problems which theories and today generally accepted knowledge had to face. Any scientific term is "a free invention of the human mind to deal better with our world" (Einstein). A scientific term (and therefore any worldview based on scientific assumptions) can only cover parts of aspects of the related issue. And it is restricted, for example, by the state of knowledge, possible observations of the environment, by the availability of terms and their meaning, etc. Therefore the state of knowledge that was considered as current has to be considered whenever we deal with historic scientific literature. When the Genesis was written, the scientific knowledge was not present to observe biochemical processes and to distinguish between different elements (in their modern sense) molecules, genes, etc., hence the story of the world being created within six days should not be considered as a literal description by our 21st century standard of knowledge; we accept this text now more as an epos about the processes than a scientific explanation of evolution.

Common people use a different language. Therefore scientists, intellectuals, politicians, etc. have to transfer their message into the language of the common people in such a way that they are able and motivated to follow the recommendations. The language of the common people is often relatively simple, therefore the messages must be adequate to their vocabulary.

"Western Medicine" is covering different states of knowledge, different worldviews and proposals to the public — depending on the (historic) period you are talking about. Unless a specific description has been added, an observer can expect that you are speaking about the actual given Western medicine of the 21st century. Such distinctions are to be taken into account in any part of the Oriental medicine too. Therefore, I understand that leading representatives of the Fudan University prefer to speak about "Chinese medicine" if they are speaking about the actual application of Chinese medicine and not to speak about "Traditional Chinese Medicine" — a medicine which is based only on the philosophy and terminology of the time of the "Yellow emperor".

2.2 The Given Situation

Western (school) medicine is often understood as a synonym for medicine based on natural sciences. But this is a simplification: In the Western medicine there are three legally accepted fields: natural science-based medicine, psychosomatic-based medicine, and the linkage to Public Health. For example, in Austria thanks to the "Law to study medicine 1972", medical psychology and social medicine are to be integrated. Therefore, MDs have to deal scientifically with the gaps between body-soul and individual-community/society. As a result medicine has to be integrated — e.g. by social medicine — into a comprehensive understanding of New Public Health. This position is effective European law (e.g. by Article 168 of the Lisboan treaty).

2.2.1 *A medicine for bodies without soul and a medicine for souls without bodies*

(Idealistic) psychosomatic medicine was developed in the late 19th and the beginning of the 20th century parallel to the medical understanding on the (materialistic) basis of modern natural science. In principle both types accept the relevance of bio-psycho-eco-socio-cultural interactions as relevant for health and illness, but without a model which allows to link these fundamentally different positions. Uexküll (1963) expressed this situation as follows: "We have two types of medicine: One medicine for bodies without souls and one for souls without bodies." Epidemiology is accepted as a sufficient linkage between them; the price that has to be paid for the lack of a model which allows to connect the materialistic and idealistic position is the shift of argumentation from causality to risk. Therefore evidence-based medicine is the actual "golden way".

There is a consequence of a fundamental shift in the relevance of philosophical argumentation within the scientific community: contrary to the 19th and early 20th century, philosophical reflections are not any more part of daily life and the educational program of many — including very efficient — natural and medical scientists. Correct scientific work seems to be given if the rules of good scientific practice (techniques in laboratory, statistics, etc.) are fulfilled. Therefore, in biology, medicine, and so on, causality is accepted if the chain of observable phenomena as a consequence of an observable stimulus can be described (though a description is not an explanation). If a natural (medical) scientist is accepting a philosophical position then it is close to positivism: Ontological positions have to be excluded as "metaphysics". Many scientists would be surprised if you were to tell them that science without a (consciously or unconsciously used) worldview (ontology) is impossible.

In some aspects the unconsciously used ontological position of Western (natural) science and medicine should be critically discussed. It can — simplified and exaggerated — be described as follows: The natural laws can be objectively detected on the basis of a material (substance-) monism by the use of empirical examination only. Therefore, there cannot be just one other model for health "science" than "(natural) science". It is necessary and sufficient to understand health and our world as a consequence of an (open) evolutionary process – essentially based on the ideas of Darwin and Mendel. *Vis vitals* and the Cartesian view are falsified. But it is accepted to understand the organism and its organs just as functional units for the purposes of the individual person. (Therefore, there is *de facto* no relevant difference to a mechanistic model.) There are unsolved questions, e.g. the body/mind problem or the gaps between individual and society, between real and virtual (e.g. economy), etc. Many scientists have the epistemologically not explainable optimistic belief that these gaps will be closed within time by the given natural scientific (positivistic) understanding. Often the tools of epistemology are seen as restricted on the technique of Popper. Many scientists believe that the bivalent (Aristotelian) logic is the only correct way of logic argumentation. There is a widespread emotional aversion against philosophical argumentations.

Even a puristic natural scientist should/could accept the preventive, promotive and curative offers of TCM as evidence-based — as a distillate of hundreds of years of systematic and critical analysis of the effects of actions and applications.

2.2.2 *(New) Public Health (PH)*

Public Health is more a political concept than a scientific one. With the advent of public health focused universities a multitude of options to expand on the current knowledge in various fundamentally different scientific disciplines has arisen. (Materialistic-based) disciplines of natural science and applications including medicine are the minority. Disciplines based on social, economic, political sciences, disciplines oriented on epidemiology, education and motivation, decision-making etc. are indispensible. But each of them has its own terminology and — usually unconsciously used — worldview. The lack of compatibility between them is an obvious problem for efficient scientific discourse. Therefore, a scientific decision about the priorities between the generally accepted targets and recommendations of the WHO-Charta is often not possible. As a consequence there is a need for a scientific fundament of PH including the concepts of WHO which allows conclusions on the level of causality. The Extended View is such a model.

2.2.3 *The debate about reproducible but unexplained phenomena*

The paper of Engel (1977) in *Science* was a milestone: he pointed out that it is not possible to confirm relevant predictions only on the basis of natural sciences about psychiatric and psychosomatic disorders. Therefore medical scientists should modify their basic concepts, but up to now they have not. This is unacceptable within the frame of scientific work. As long as there is no correct reaction medical science can no longer be accepted as a science. Engel proposed the need of a so-called "bio-psycho-social model". It should be possible to deduce it on the basis of the General System Theory and of a hierarchical follow-up of evolutionary-based subsystems, but up to now this proposal is more a vision than an applicable model. The theory seems plausible since system theory is helpful within the different subsystems (e.g. of cells, individuals, societies) but it does not allow a linkage between the subsystems due to epistemological reasons; the terminologies which are used in the different subsystem cannot be transferred from one to the other subsystem. So the bio-psycho-social model is generally accepted but used just on the basis of epidemiology.

Recently incompatibilities even within the traditional natural scientific disciplines stimulated growing critical discussions about the dogmatic use of the given natural scientific paradigm. Examples are the consequences of the fundamentally changed understanding of the determinative power of genes with respect to, e.g., epigenetic and proteomic effects. Therefore, the number of scientists who are discussing the need of an extended view of evolution is increasing. Typical representatives are Jablonka and her colleagues from MIT. They discuss the need to distinguish between four types of evolution (Jablonka and Lamb, 2006). Another example is a remarkable initiative by the so-called Altenberg 16, a group of internationally well-known scientists - primarily from biology – who met 2009 at the institute of the late Nobel Laureate Konrad Lorenz. They put up for discussion the fact that selection cannot be the only principle to explain the evolutionary progress scientifically (Mazur, 2010).

An underestimated discussion is ongoing about how to handle the incompatibilities within the different paradigms in physics and chemistry, which can be understood as an implicit discussion about immaterial aspects: So Nobel laureate H.J. Muller proposed to introduce a so-called "heterocatalytic power" to explain why genes can stimulate the reproduction of another structure different from their own (Muller, 1922). And Nobel laureate Heisenberg proposed to attribute to the quanta a "*potentia*", which should explain the ability of genes to select individually between options within borders by natural given laws (Heisenberg, 1958). Einstein created a new worldview on the basis of a natural philosophy; because of this he received (as the only natural scientist) the highest honor of philosophy: a volume in "The library of the living philosophers" was dedicated to his work (Schilpp, 1949). He developed techniques to handle given incompatibilities between indispensible theories, e.g. the theories of Newton and Maxwell. He used these philosophical techniques and his new paradigm just as tools. Doing so he was able to create the Relativity Theories. This demonstrates the power of his ideas to link theories which are helpful but formerly were not to be linked on a causal level. Therefore, I have used Einstein's ideas to link the different health-related disciplines. Maybe this should be discussed with respect to Chinese Medicine as well.

2.3 Some Remarks on the Philosophy of Einstein

For Einstein the crucial problem was the incompatibility of the understanding of movement according to the mechanics of Newton and the electromagnetism of Maxwell. They seem to exclude each other according to the third sentence of Aristotle: If one assumption excludes another one totally, only one of them can be right, the other one must be wrong and there is no third solution. Newton is teaching us: A scientific statement about the movement of a star can be only correct if you integrate the position and the movement of the observer. Maxwell is teaching us: A scientific statement about the movement of the light of this star can only be correct if you do

NOT integrate the position and the movement of the observer. In consequence a correct physicist would have to choose: To accept Newton and refuse Maxwell or vice versa. This was inacceptable for Einstein: Both theories are indispensible (like natural science-based medicine and psychosomatic and social-oriented medicine are). His solution was that the contradiction was not the nature. The simplifications which are used by the terminologies of Newton and Maxwell are incompatible. Einstein made the conclusions:

(1) We cannot have an ideal "objective" knowledge of the world. Any scientific term (and any scientific law, theory, etc.) is a "free invention of the human mind" and belongs to another category than that for what they stand for. Therefore scientists have to create terms and/or have to modify their meaning if the phenomena cannot be explained or distinctly communicated with the given terminology.
(2) Such new terms can only be established if they are backed by empirical data. The natural scientific part of the creation of the Relativity Theories was the creation of applicable adjustments of the formulas of Newton and Maxwell. But this was only possible with a modification of the worldview: quanta are able to move themselves actively according to Einstein. The objects are moved passively in the world of Newton.
(3) The "real progress" in science is to be expected by the use of so-called "Real Theories": This is a special type of meta-theories which allows to link theories which have not been linked before because of the incompatibility of the used terminologies and ontology. This can be done by modification of the meaning of terms which are used with different meanings in the (former) incommensurate theories. The invention of the new meaning has to cover the needs of all theories which should be linked by the new "real theory". Therefore, the scientist has to think about "what is behind" the content actually used (e.g. of movement) — so that the applications (e.g. for mechanics as well as for electromagnetism) can be understood as a special application of the "more basic definition". In the terminology of set theory you can say: Theories which have been before distinct ground sets (e.g. mechanics and electromagnetism) can now be integrated as

subsets in a more fundamental ground set (Relativity Theories). Therefore, it is correct to use the theories as usual for the typical problems. It is only in cases dealing with different theories covered within the "Real Theory" that the terminology and techniques of the "Real Theory" allow additional power, and should be used just for such cases. Therefore, it is obvious that the Real Theory does not falsify an existing (correct) theory. The existing theory is still fully functional to solve the issues for which it was originally developed.

2.4 Application of the Proposal of Einstein on the Extended View

I used these techniques to develop my "Extended View" which can be understood as a "bio-psycho-socio-eco-cultural model."

The basic assumption is: There are scientific disciplines for nearly all health-related aspects, but there are gaps due to their different ontologies and incompatible terminology. If we had just one theoretical framework to integrate all the different sectoral disciplines then the incompatibilities would disappear. Einstein's technique for Real Theories gives hope that such a model could be realized.

I discuss three types of incompatibilities:

(1) incompatibilities caused by a different monistic ontology (materialism vs. idealism);
(2) to accept invisible abilities of the interacting objects for causality or not; and
(3) incompatibilities in the contents of terms. In this paper I use just the term "evolution". There are different meanings, e.g. between biology, cosmology, linguistic.

2.4.1 *Compatibility of different monistic ontologies*

Substance-dualistic models (e.g. the Cartesian model) have been falsified. But *substance-monistic* models are accepted by everyone. Natural sciences accept a materialistic substance monism. Non-natural sciences use an idealistic substance monism. Both seem to exclude each other — with good reasons. Science should restrict itself on what is relevant to handle the given problem adequately. For example, it is not helpful to integrate the materialistic aspect of money (the quality of paper) for the explanation of modifications in the exchange rate between Euro and Dollar. And there are cases which can be handled sufficiently just with a materialistic monism, e.g. to calculate the speed of a falling stone. If you accept that the decision for an idealistic or materialistic position depends on the problem that should be solved as easily as possible, then it would not be a problem to accept a neutral substance monistic position that accepts evolutionary processes in general and select the appropriate choice according to the actual problem. Therefore the exclusion would result only if the ontological position is assumed as an objective statement about the nature of the world. But we will use philosophical positions just as tools to deal more appropriate with our daily life problems.

2.4.2 *Compatibility of the levels of argumentation*

There is a relevant imbalance between the levels of argumentation in classical physics and chemistry on one hand, and all the other health-related sciences on the other: In physics and chemistry you accept invisible influences (e.g. fields, forces, power) to explain observable effects upon the single case. And thanks to these abilities we can explain why an individual is able to be active and reactive on an energetical level, e.g. to move a picture from one side of the wall to the other. It is different in other disciplines dealing with, e.g. life, emotional, cognitive or intellectual activities. We cannot explain with a similar chain of argumentation why a person can learn, e.g. to distinct different faces in a picture with more options of interpretation. Such processes are also relevant for the understanding of differences in the understanding of similar situations between elderly and youngsters, between different cultures but also for the understanding of happiness, wellbeing, etc.

Natural scientists exclude such questions since *vis vitalis* and the Cartesian dualism were falsified in agreement with a positivistic position, but they do not dispute the existence of life-related, emotional, cognitive and intellectual abilities. They delegate the answers to other scientific disciplines. But exclusion is not a scientific solution for the problem. Therefore, a model is needed which is compatible with the falsification of substance dualisms and *vis vitalis* on one hand and the fact of immaterial aspects of daily life on the other.

We postulate just one invisible substance which allows to be effective. We call it "*potentia*"— with respect to Aristotle and Heisenberg; this is a substance-monistic position. According to the principle to start as simply as possible, we have attributed to the most basic actors just two types of effects: one for the materialistic, and one for the idealistic aspects. But both are the expression of just one substance. We can compare the situation with a coin of gold, e.g. a Chinese Panda in your hand. The whole coin consists of just one substance: gold. This substance enables to form two different sides: one with the panda and one with the temple of heaven. But you can only see one side at the same time. The decision for the position of the coin in your hand excludes you from observing the other side at the same time. You cannot observe the bottom side if you observe the upper side. This should express the consequence of limitation (conservational laws). According to N. Bohr we attribute to *potentia* two aspects that are complementary, which means to be able to modify relations on an energetical/materialistic basis or on an informational/idealistic basis. If you transfer complementarity into a dynamic process you can call it "polarity".

The two aspects of *potentia* are related to each other, so the evolutionary level of the morphological structure defines the level on which can be dealt with information. But the evolutionary level to deal with information limits the possibilities to use morphological structures; therefore, persons are not monkeys, monkeys not amoebas and amoebas not crystals, but they all use *potentia* to modify relations within time and space as well as within meaning — each on its "evolutionary level".

The term covering the ability to modify on an energetical/materialistic basis is well known — it is "energy" (according to the meaning given by modern physicists and chemists) There is no internationally used term for the complementary ability.

According to the recommendation of Einstein we had to introduce a term for this ability to deal with immaterial aspects. I call this ability "discrimination ability". It enables us to, for example, attribute information to matter. I had to characterize the ability for empirical testing. One assumption was that the conservational laws should be in effect.

Therefore the available capacity of this ability is limited. A consequence of this assumption is that any healing and growing process needs an adequate amount of such a — restricted available — ability. With an adequate amount of this ability, homeostasis is only to be expected, therefore we should expect an increase in the severity of symptoms and the mortality rate if additional demands for adaptation are given. We could confirm this prediction, e.g. in the changing of mortality distribution of victims of Hiroshima and Nagasaki with identical loads of radioactivity but different demands to deal additional to the radioactivity with healing processes, physical burdens, growing or the consequences of aging. This contribution was selected as the Thomas Kuhn — Hope for the Future for a sustainable world — Award 2004 (Kofler, 2005).

2.4.3 *Compatibility of different meanings of the term evolution*

The "extended view" should cover all health-related aspects with respect to their occurrence within the evolutionary process. The "oldest" are the quanta: Without quanta no vitamin D etc.

According to Einstein, I had to invent characteristics "behind" the quanta. These "free inventions of the human mind" should allow the deduction of the autopoiesis of quanta. The assumptions about quanta should be the "ground set" for the "extended view" as basis for a follow-up from the autopoiesis of quanta to the autopoiesis of human persons, societies and culture. The invention should allow the inclusion of the health-related aspects of different former distinct theories as subsets, but there is a fundamental problem: it is not sufficient to only describe when evolutionary progress has taken place (as is done for example in cosmological models), but the health relevant aspects of "evolution" have to be deduced as well.

There is consent between scientists about evolution that all the time more theoretical options for modifications are given than the finally realized option, therefore there is a need to explain the reason for the section between them. Also, there is consent between scientists that the given evolutionary processes cannot/should not be explained neither with a machine model or intelligent design nor with an indispensible permanent influence from outside our universe. But during any period of the evolutionary progress nothing else was present than the actually given entities with their abilities. If you agree with these positions then you agree implicitly with the conclusion, that the actually existing entities and their relationships are sufficient and necessary causes for the decision between the different options for realization and as the sufficient and necessary reason for the realization/creation of the "New" (the emergent). We cannot explain "to observe the actual situation, to evaluate the options to react to it" as well as "decision making" and "to initiate a realization" just with materialism. And we cannot explain "realization" just with idealism. This fits with the invention of "the polarity of *potentia*" and its modifiability within the borders of the laws of conservation.

This model includes implicitly the assumption that the actor has an individual range of freedom, but is restricted, e.g., by the environmental given, the reached evolutionary level, the relevance to be in consent and especially to keep the reached level of evolutionary existence. The consequences of the given borders can be predicted — the way constraint individuals are using the free range cannot. This "range of freedom for individual decisions" allows us to explain the emergent phenomena and that the occurrence of these phenomena cannot be predicted — neither in time nor in space. Therefore, the occurrence of an adequate environment can be a necessary prerequisite for the emergence but not sufficient for the beginning of any evolutionary progress. We should expect the following follow-up — but just in the cases in which the actor is able to observe and evaluate the environment, knows about its options and the possibilities to modify them: The "environmental offer" has to be "seen by an individual actor, as everybody can see it", but it has "to be recognized as nobody before has recognized it". Then the actor had to select between the different possibilities to react and has to select the adequate one. So the emergent is realized the first time. But if the progress is not used by many others, then the possible evolutionary win goes lost with the extinction of the inventor. The spreading of the emergent is to be expected if the inventor is willing to share the gain/success with others. And this is not enough: Usually the use of an emergent application is linked to an additional restriction of options and therefore to a loss of freedom. It must be conclusive for additional users, that the gain/success is bigger than the loss and that the spreading of the emergent phenomenon within a wider community does not reduce the individual surplus chance for success/gain unacceptably. But this type of evolutionary progress can take place within a short time.

2.4.4 *Open aspects*

The follow-up of steps from the invention of an emergent option to a widespread evolutionary success/change deals with cases in which the actor knows what kind of functions he can use directly or by modifying. It describes effectively the creation of "new", e.g. by humans in a community and/or society, but it does not explain the relevance of genetics, epigenetics and proteomics for such human processes. It is state of knowledge: Even a person who has learned all the new data of epigenetics etc. is not able to influence voluntarily its genetic "book of life" for a more appropriate answer neither for physiological needs nor for emotional, cognitive or intellectual challenges. This "book of life" is a prerequisite which enables the person to perform a given variety of activities but within strict borders. Is this an incompatibility with the state of knowledge in biology and inacceptable for a linkage of the "extended view" with the evolutionary theory or with genetics, epigenetics and proteomics? I do not think so.

(1) The "Extended View" as well as the related biological disciplines accept that the genetic treasure is such a "book of life". It is not possible to answer neither with the help of the "Extended View" nor with one of the related biological disciplines who can read this book. Therefore, there is no incompatibility with the given sectoral disciplines.
(2) There is no discussion about the possibility that an existing but formerly not relevant morphological option can be helpful and lifesaving under changing conditions. There is no contradiction that the chemical structure of DNA can be modified by external influences on the basis of probability and that the information that is linked with them will be changed. Yet there is no discussion that even this change of information has to be evaluated, but there is no answer who is doing this — neither by the biological disciplines nor within the "Extended View". Both have to accept the result of the evaluation and have to attribute it to the "complex actor".

(3) The actual state of knowledge about biological evolution usually accepts as its starting point the existence of life and explains the morphology and biological processes with genes. This is understood as based on a materialistic monism. The — simplified — only accepted mechanisms for evolution are probability of mutation, selection of the appropriate mutations and the selection of the sexual partners with respect to optimize the genetic pool. Is this really a "pure materialistic" position? We accept that a human person is not able to know anything about genes (if the person has not learned about it at school). But the female animals should be able to deal (instinctively?) with the intention to optimize the genes of their offspring. Male animals fight with other males to give their genes to as many offspring as possible. We also know, for example, that different male monkeys kill the offspring of their precursors because of this reason. Is this really a materialistic position? Such an "ancient inborn based instinct" would need an ancient fundament about an ancient possibility to use genes to extend offers for morphological realizations. But on the evolutionary highly differentiated level of mammals and monkeys such an "inborn instinct" could explain easier the selection of impressive observables then the "conscious-like" selection of sexual partners with "better" genetic pools. These arguments fit to the phenomena and to the conclusion that even the position of modern biology is not to be understood on the basis of a "pure materialism" only.

(4) The "Extended View" offers a proposal for the autopoiesis of life by an extended use of morphological structures to extend the memory about possible realizations. The model makes it plausible that "higher multicellulars" are organized by cell-systems which cannot have the full information about the possibilities to modify the genetic code — because of their differentiation in the function between different types of cells and cell systems. Such restrictions are to be expected especially after the autopoiesis of emotion, intellectual and cognitive options. Yet living beings on such a high level should use additionally to the biological forces and weapons more and more emotional, intellectual and cognitive options to realize their intentions including their (emotional and social) survival. The morphological structure for that is based on the genetic code, but these structures seem to be nearly

identical in principle in humans for several thousand years already. Therefor the genetically based fundamentals seem to be more or less given in any healthy human being. The difference in the adequate use is more restricted by the modules of neuronal nets in the brain and their use: To decide to accept one solution or the opposite, and to realize it or not. These decisions, which are relevant to understand the human individual as a social being, have the genetic code as a prerequisite. There are relevant reasons not to accept that they define the individual intellectual or logical decisions.

(5) The most relevant argument that the given lack in linkage to genetically based health effects are not incompatibilities between the intentions of the creation of the "Extended View", is that there are no applications needed to deal better with genetically based diseases or health promotion.

2.4.5 *Further information*

In this paper I can only present the application of Einstein´s theory for our modified epistemological technique. Some aspects about its transfer to the "Extended View" and the additional power for (social) medicine, Public Health and sustainability, which has been published. Key aspects can be looked up in the Sechenov Honor Lecture 2004 (Kofler, 2005).

2.5 Remarks on the Chinese Medical Model

Any frame of science is a "free invention of the human mind" (Einstein). Therefore, different scientific understandings may emerge. No theory is without restrictions for its applicability. Therefore, it is always helpful to think about other frameworks, their potentials and their restrictions — even as an instrument to see clearer the restrictions of the personally preferred framework, especially according to the topic of this paper: to respect underestimated aspects, e.g. of the implicit fundamentals of Western medicine models.

There are familiarities in the Western and Eastern self-understanding. Maybe some of the latter are not as highly regarded in Western Medicine as they should be, but surely they deserve further attention.

- Chinese medicine is focusing on balance — Western Medicine accepts homoeostasis
- The diagnostic methods in TCM are based on inspection, smelling and auscultation, palpation and personal communication. Maybe these aspects could be re-intensified but are more and more suppressed by the technical instruments to collect data.
- Both models accept a holistic view including the relevance of the external surrounding (environmental, social, etc.)
- Both views accept a three-column-model of health: curative, preventive and promotive aspects, but with fundamental, nearly opposite differences in emphasis. Promotive aspects are nearly neglected in many Western teaching programs in relation to the dominant curative aspects.

Different aspects of the scientific self-understanding of Chinese Medicine are focused on similar aspects like the "Extended view" and the proposal of Engel:

(1) Substance monism with a plurality of qualities.
(2) Permanent process with liberties but within given borders.
(3) Dynamic polarity of qualities (to enable materialistic and idealistic effects). This seems to be in strong agreement with the complementarity in nature (N. Bohr), not only to explain the restriction which is inherent to any empirical technique but also to the consequence of a dynamic shift in the use of options.
(4) Relevance of the understanding of the organism as an entity itself which should be balanced — with the consequence to enable the individual to use the organism for purposes of a person.
(5) The relevance to be in balance with different parts of the given (social, cultural, ecological) world.
(6) Chinese Medical books often offer introductions into the ontological and epistemological fundamentals of the application (e.g. *Healthy Aging* (Leung, 2011), *Der ältere Patient in der chinesischen Medizin* (Noll, 2006), and *Handout for Austrian Students* (Wang, 2011).

Therefore we should expect a stimulating process if we listen carefully and with respect to the experiences which are given in the different parts of the world. And this should allow us to improve the offers for health, wellbeing and competence in the actually elderly and the actually young generation — the elderly of tomorrow and the partners of the elderly of today.

References

Darwin, C. (1871) *The Origin of Species*. Appleton, New York.

Descartes, R. and Wohlers, C. (2005) *Die Prinzipien der Philosophie*. Meiner, Hamburg.

Du Bois-Reymond, E.H. (1882) *Ueber die Grenzen des Naturerkennens. Die Sieben Weltraethsel*. Veit, Leipzig.

Engel, G.L. (1977) The need for a new medical model: a challenge for biomedicine. *Science* **196**, 129–136.

Heisenberg, W. (1958) *Physics and Philosophy. The Revolution in Modern Science*. Harper & Row, New York.

Jablonka, E. and Lamb, M.J. (2006) *Evolution in Four Dimensions*. MIT Press, Cambridge, MA.

Kofler, W. (2005) In: *14th Sechenov Lectures* (eds.) Russian Academy of Science *et al.* International Academy of Science H&E, Moscow, pp. 2–68.

Kuhn, T. (1962) *The Structure of Scientific Revolution*. University of Chicago Press, Chicago.

Leung, P.C. (2011) *Healthy Aging*. World Scientific, New Jersey.

Mazur, S. (2010) *The Altenberg 16. An Expose of the Evolution Industry*. North Atlantic, Berkeley, California.

Muller, H.J. (1922) Variation due to change in the individual gene. *Am. Nat.* **56**, 32–50.

Noll, A.A. (2006) *Der aeltere Patient in der Chinesischen Medizin. Gesund alt Werden, Alterskrankheiten Vorbeugen und Behandeln*. Elsevier, Urban und Fischer, Muenchen/Jena.

Schilpp, P.A. (1949) *Albert Einstein: Philosopher-Scientist*. Evanston, New York.

Schmidt, W. (2004) Personal communication between Walter Schmidt, one of the followers of Roux on the cathedra for anatomy and embryology at the University of Innsbruck, and Walter Kofler, Innsbruck.

Uexkuell, T. (1963) *Grundfragen der Psychosomatischen Medizin*. Rowohlt, Reinbek bei Hamburg.

Wang, Y. (2011) *Handout for Austrian Students*. Beijing University of Chinese Medicine, Beijing.

Chapter 3

The Hong Kong Cadenza Philosophy

Ruby Yu and Jean Woo

Abstract

Hong Kong is a city in the Special Administrative Region of China with a population of seven million living in a space of 1104 square kilometers. It has the longest life expectancy for men in the world while for women, life expectancy is second only to Japan. By 2036 those aged 65 and over are projected to form one quarter of the total population. This demographic change has raised concerns regarding the anticipated increase in burden of chronic diseases and disability as well as worsening mental health in our society. To counterbalance this somewhat pessimistic view, the CADENZA project was started in 2006, to highlight how our society can meet these challenges in a positive way, emphasizing the person-centered perspective and importance of the non-medical approach. This project was initiated by the Hong Kong Jockey Club Charities Trust, partnered by tertiary institutions and non-government organizations, and consists of four major components: public education training, community projects, and leadership training. Under this program a community center (Jockey club CADENZA Hub) has been established, for the soon-to-be old as well as the elderly, their carers and volunteers, adopting Eastern and Western philosophies in a trans-disciplinary, trans-cultural and holistic approach. The services provided by the Hub broadly responds to the three stages of the aging process: health promotion, health maintenance and prevention of decline, applying behavioral modification principles; optimizing control and maintaining function for those with chronic diseases emphasizing self-management techniques; and providing physical and psychological support for those with frailty and their carers using a case management approach. The center provides a venue for further downstream diffusion of programs that have been developed and evaluated to meet service needs from the users' perspective to be integrated into current service provisions.

Keywords: CADENZA; Person-centered perspective; Non-medical approach; Philosophy; Aging process.

3.1 Introduction

According to a population projection by the Census and Statistics Department in 2007, the population in Hong Kong will be on an aging trend, with the elderly population (aged 65 and above) projected to rise from 12% in 2006 to 26% in 2036. In 2006, the life expectancy at birth is 79.5 years and 85.6 years for males and females respectively, and is projected to rise to 82.7 years for males and 88.3 years for females by 2036. This translates to a disproportionately large elderly population made up mostly of females with a high elderly dependency ratio (Census and Statistics Department of Kong Kong, 2007). This demographic change has raised concerns regarding the anticipated increase in burden of chronic diseases and disability as well as worsening mental health in our society.

The number of people with impairment and dependency will increase significantly over the next 20 years, which poses serious social and economic challenges for our society. There will be practical considerations such as the availability of community support, demand on social services and health care services, quality and availability of family and community caregivers, quality and availability of residential homes, and so on. There are also considerable drains on public resources and a greater demand for social and medical services, straining both the health and social care systems.

There is an increasing amount of evidence relating to the gains from better joint working between the health and social care systems (Johri *et al.*, 2003). The government and many non-government organizations (NGOs) have engaged in different aspects of aging and elderly care, but there still exists many documented misconceptions amongst the public as well as professionals with many gaps in services. In view of the challenges Hong Kong may face for its aging population, the CADENZA: A Jockey Club Initiative for Seniors was conceived by the Hong Kong Jockey Club (HKJC) Charities Trust in 2006 to highlight how our society can meet these challenges in a positive way, emphasizing the person-centered perspective and the importance of the non-medical approach.

CADENZA: A Jockey Club Initiative for Seniors (www.cadenza.org.hk) is a HK $380 million project, that engages partners from different institutions, organizations and professions, and has the potential to cut across traditional barriers and initiate positive changes towards a more elder-friendly Hong Kong through professional education, training, raising public awareness, and supporting community demonstration projects, underpinned by evidence-based practice. The project partners are the Faculty of Social Sciences of The University of Hong Kong and Faculty of Medicine of The Chinese University of Hong Kong.

CADENZA is an acronym for "**C**elebrate their **A**ccomplishments; **D**iscover their **E**ffervescence and **N**ever-ending **Z**est as they **A**ge." In classical music, a "CADENZA" is an extended virtuosic section, usually near the end of a movement in a concerto. The word is used figuratively to describe the apex of one's life and the celebration of a lifetime's accomplishments.

3.2 The Principles

There are seven principles underpinning all activities and services development of the CADENZA project. They are:

(1) to recognize that choices and priorities of the individual are at the center of planning and delivery;
(2) to recognize the importance of non-medical factors:
  - health promotion and maintenance, by applying behavioral modification principles
  - self-management of chronic conditions
  - physical and psychological support in frailty;

(3) to raise the level of health literacy regarding aging issues in the community through health education, and to improve self-management and empowerment;
(4) to highlight concern about social inclusion, volunteerism, and personhood of the elderly, particularly at the end of life;
(5) to develop community models, plan and provide services and assessments based in the community to attract participation;
(6) to involve the soon-to-be old as well as elderly, carers, and volunteers in assessment and services planning; and
(7) to adopt Eastern and Western philosophies in a trans-disciplinary, trans-cultural and holistic approach.

3.3 Project Vision

The CADENZA project aims to contribute to shaping an elder friendly environment in Hong Kong from the perspective of an individual, covering not only social, physical and psychological health components, but also including the physical living environment from home to neighborhood to the city as a whole.

3.4 Four Major Components of the Cadenza Project

CADENZA project has four major components: (1) public education, (2) training, (3) community, and (4) leadership training. Through these four components, various projects, activities, and services were organized to create an elder-friendly community in Hong Kong. Detailed information relating to the four major components and their achievements are described in the following sections.

3.4.1 *Public education*

A series of research activities has been carried out to gather data and evidence that informs the overall theme of promoting an elder-friendly environment in the broad sense, and to provide the rationale for the public education program, as well as all the other components of CADENZA. Six themes were identified, including (1) health promotion and maintenance, (2) health and social services, (3) living environment, (4) legal and financial issues, (5) quality of life and quality of dying, and (6) ageism and age disparities. These six themes of CADENZA have been covered in several large scale public education programs to achieve wide penetration of the positive aging messages.

3.4.1.1 *CADENZA 18-district program*

It was a citywide public education initiative jointly organized with Radio Television Hong Kong (RTHK) Radio 5. The program ran for 18 months from January 2009 to July 2010 aiming to revolutionize the ways people view and care for the elderly, to equip the soon-to-be-old with knowledge contributing to active and positive aging, and to highlight topics pertaining to positive aging to residents of Hong Kong's 18 districts, having regard to specific local characteristics. A total of 15 events have been organized in different districts, with 6500 invited participants and passers-by of all ages. More than 90% of the participants found the events helpful in correcting their misconceptions and enhancing their knowledge on aging.

3.4.1.2 *CADENZA TV series*

Co-produced with RTHK, a Television Broadcasts Limited (TVB) Jade (a TV channel in Hong Kong) TV series comprising of ten half-hour episodes prepared for the challenges posed by an aging population, hence promoting active aging and projecting a positive public image of the seniors. Each episode carried positive aging messages expressed through challenges encountered by the characters involved. The TV series was developed alongside the six themes of CADENZA and has won two international awards including a Certificate of Merit in the 45th Chicago Intercom Competition 2009 for the episode on dementia and a Certificate of Merit in the 2010 Hugo Television Awards for the whole series. An average of 1.2 million viewers was recorded for the TV series with an average TV rating of 19 points.

3.4.1.3 *CADENZA press conference*

A series of six press conferences taking the six themes of CADENZA has been organized, with the aim to arouse public awareness of different issues related to the elderly and to announce research findings. These press conferences were: (1) Does very hot weather warning reduce mortality among elderly people in Hong Kong? (July 2008), (2) Can we avoid spending the last part of our lives in old age homes? (September 2008), (3) Challenges of population aging Part I: How well are seniors in Hong Kong doing? (November 2008), (4) New attitude and new direction in elderly care (February 2009), (5) Challenges of population aging on disease trends and burden Part II: Diabetes (May 2009), and (6) Challenges of population aging on disease trends and burden Part III: Dementia (April 2010). These press conferences were covered by six radio interviews and more than 55 local media.

3.4.1.4 *CADENZA Symposium*

A series of four symposiums taking four themes of CADENZA has been organized, with the aim to provide a platform annually where policy makers, practitioners, researchers and the public can share experiences and exchange new insights in understanding aging issues. These four themes were: (1) Preparing for an Elder Friendly Hong Kong (January 2007), (2) Successful Aging (October 2008), (3) Primary Care and Older Persons — Key to Medical and Social Integration (October 2009), and (4) Age-Friendly World Cities and Environment (October 2010). Each symposium was attended by more than 400 participants and over 90% of the participants evaluated the symposium as useful.

3.4.1.5 *Other activities*

CADENZA has also organized other activities to raise public awareness of the aging issue. Healthy aging carnival, a one-day Elder Friendly Hong Kong Educational Fair has been held in the School of Public Health, Prince of Wales Hospital in 2007. Over 1200 people attended and many of them were members from elderly centers all over Hong Kong together with their families. A CADENZA website (www.cadenza.org.hk) has been developed which provides the philosophy underlying the project, information on all the activities, downloadable power point presentations on all press conferences and symposia, and links to RTHK radio CADENZA programs. Articles about CADENZA project were also published in different media including Hong Kong Economic Times, Ming Pao: Elderly Day 2009 Supplement, The University of Hong Kong and The Chinese University of Hong Kong Faculty Newsletters, as well as CADENZA E-Newsletter.

3.4.2 ***Training***

The CADENZA Training Program, led by The Nethersole School of Nursing, The Chinese University of Hong Kong, commenced in May 2008. It is a citywide interdisciplinary project designed to provide general and professional education in gerontology. It aims to provide training of skills and the way people view and treat the seniors they serve. Target groups include health and social care professionals, frontline workers involved in elderly work, informal and family carers, and the general public. Core part of the training program is the web-based training material complemented by practical experience and public seminars. Program activities include online courses, seminars, workshops, clinical attachments, district-based seminar, courses and self-help groups, clinical visits, carnivals, radio programs, roadshows, as well as educational leaflets and booklets. These activities involving 45 non-NGOs have been run in 18 districts in Hong Kong. Over 26,000 people participated and over 13,000 people have been trained, including nurses, social workers, occupational therapists, physiotherapists, management executives and the general public.

A comment from Ms. Bella Luk, Executive Director of Helping Hand: "Initially, I questioned about the usefulness of CADENZA Training Program as there have already been so many in the market… After reading carefully about the course outline and the teaching format, I decided to go for it. In the past months, I took the online courses, joined the clinical visits, attended seminars and workshops... I am so happy that all these activities give me an eye opening look into elderly care… I highly recommend CADENZA training program."

3.4.3 *Community projects*

CADENZA community projects are innovative and sustainable service models which cover all the mentioned principles to cope with the changing needs of seniors, especially in achieving seamless interface and collaboration among various sectors and mobilizing untapped community resources. Each project has an evidence-based research component to measure outcome and validate the effectiveness of the delivery model. It is hoped that these models will be taken up as regular services in the community provided by other exiting service providers, including government and various NGOs. Six community projects have been funded including: (1) Jockey Club CADENZA Hub, (2) Chronic Disease Self-Management Program, (3) Elder-Friendly Employment Practice, (4) Health-Social Partnership Transitional Care Model for Post-discharged Elderly, (5) Transitional Care for Stroke Patients, and (6) Elder at PEACE. These six projects are covered in more details in the following sections.

3.4.3.1 *Jockey club CADENZA hub*

Worldwide, the response to population aging in developed countries is the development of community care. Currently in Hong Kong, NGOs have various constraints in starting self-financing services as they are subvented by the government. Hence the Hong Kong Jockey Club is in a position to pioneer a model without such constraints, with the eventual aim for the model to be adopted by existing service providers.

The Jockey Club Cadenza Hub located in Tai Po Fu Shin Estate is one of the innovative community projects aiming at improving quality of care and quality of life for older persons in Hong Kong. The Jockey Club Cadenza Hub, established since September 2009, is an integrated primary health and social care center managed by The Chinese University of Hong Kong and a team of multi-disciplinary health care professionals for the soon-to-be old as well as the elderly, their carers and volunteers.

The Hub adopts Eastern and Western philosophies in a trans-disciplinary, trans-cultural and holistic approach to promote primary health and social care. Its conceptual model broadly responses the three stages of the aging process: (1) health promotion, health maintenance and prevention of decline, applying behavioral modification principles; (2) optimizing control and maintaining function for those with chronic diseases emphasizing self-management techniques; and (3) providing physical and psychological support for those with frailty and their carers using a case management approach.

The Hub provides adult day care service for people with functional disability and dementia, and a wide spectrum of wellness, lifestyle medication, health maintenance programs, as well as on-site co-location services, Traditional Chinese Medicine, audiology, and optometric assessment. It also provides a venue for further downstream diffusion of programs that have been developed and evaluated to meet service needs from the user's perspective to be integrated into current service provisions.

Below are some of the features of the Hub that distinctive from all other existing community centers: The services are designed from user's perspective, which are comprehensive and multidisciplinary in nature. It provides flexible programs and products based on local evaluation of effectiveness for health and psychological benefits. It emphasizes raising health literacy and empowerment and all services are provided in a community setting in a social context, which includes health aspects but it is not medically dominant. It is also self-sustaining, with partners from local GPs, NGOs in the community as well as Hospital Authority of Hong Kong.

The Hub has also placed a lot of importance on dissemination and knowledge sharing. The concept of one-stop services covering the whole spectrum from soon-to-be old to those with frailty has been discussed in various discussion forums and seminars and it is being considered for the Senior Residences Projects developed by the Hong Kong Housing Society and Hong Kong Council of Social Service, which would possibly lead to a greater impact in the society.

A comment from Chief Officer of Hong Kong Council of Social Service (Elderly Services): "The one-stop service model is a demonstration of the elderly service development I am so touched that in the CADENZA Hub, the caregivers in particular those older women are going to benefit in a holistic way. Their physical and social status would be enhanced through the meaningful engagement in the Hub... it is a pleasure to learn from you and your staff."

3.4.3.2 *Chronic disease self-management program (CDSMP)*

In partnering with the Salvation Army and Shatin Hospital, the Chronic Disease Self-Management Program is another community project to help older people to manage their chronic disease(s) so as to prevent avoidable hospitalizations and minimize their reliance on medical service. Over 450 elderly people participated and they showed improvement in better self-management behaviour, improved self-efficacy in managing their diseases, enhanced health status, reduced incidence of depressive symptoms, pain and discomfort, and decline in health care utilization. Results were shared with the public in a seminar cum press conference. The effectiveness of the program was welcomed by social and health care sectors.

3.4.3.3 *Elder-friendly employment practice*

In partnering with the Hong Kong Society for the Aged, the Elder-Friendly Employment Practice framework was developed to attract and retain older workers staying in work, and to give them a sense of inclusion and recognition in the community. More than 900 older people participated in a study carried out by CADENZA research team to identify their needs to remain in the workforce. The findings have been shared with the public in a symposium cum press conference in May 2010. To enhance the employability of active retirees, a STAR program also commenced in April 2009. One hundred older people have participated in the training program. The results of these programs are to arouse community discussion. Currently some major organizations are also focusing on this area, including the government's Efficiency Unit of the Hong Kong government. The Hong Kong Shanghai Bank has also started a very good elder employment program.

3.4.3.4 *Health-social partnership transitional care model for post-discharged elderly*

In partnership with the Salvation Army, Queen Elizabeth Hospital and the Hong Kong Polytechnic University, a 28-day comprehensive and intensive transitional care program was developed to reduce avoidable hospital readmission. A total of 638 patients have been recruited, and 159 volunteers recruited from NGOs have been trained to help run the educational and behavioral modification programs. The results of the project have been shared with the public in a symposium cum press conference in July 2010. This model has been taken up as regular services in Queen Elizabeth Hospital and has been also integrated to the discharge program of Hospital Authority of Hong Kong.

3.4.3.5 *Transitional care for stroke patients*

In partnering with Hong Kong Sheng Kung Hui Welfare Council, a transitional care program for stroke patients has been organized to provide an integrated and multi-dimensional stroke rehabilitation program to help maximize stroke patients' potential for independent living and prevent avoidable hospital readmission and to fill the existing service gap of providing more care options for those who can afford to pay. There were 350 enquiries about the services, and 79 site visits have been arranged for

210 invited guests, including general practioners, nurses as well as representatives from NGOs and private hospitals. Twenty-six clients have been admitted with a total 2312 patient days and an average length of stay of 89 days. Articles about the program were also published in different media including Oriental Daily News and Taiwan Magazine.

3.4.3.6 *Elder at PEACE*

In partnering with Hong Kong Christian Service, a district wide program is being provided in Kwai Tsing, Hong Kong, where prevalence of elder abuse is high, involving District Council members along with Social Welfare Department and NGO stakeholders. This district-wide program aims to provide immediate and medium to long-term assistance and services to victims of elder abuse and related parties, to establish a multidisciplinary district-based practice model for screening, identification, assessment, intervention and follow-up, to furnish an evidence-based intervention model for abused elders and their carers, and to raise public awareness on elder abuse and foster elder justice. The program has commenced in May 2010. It is hoped that the model will spread to other districts and be taken up as regular community services provided by NGOs.

3.4.2 *Leadership training*

In view of an aging society and the lack of interest in gerontology in Hong Kong among the academic sector, the CADENZA Fellowship training program, modeled after a similar program funded by The John A. Hartford Foundation in the USA, could produce good leaders who would champion the cause of older people, help shape future government policy, and form a network of support to train the next generation of geriatric social and health care workers. Since 2007, 30 faculty members from various tertiary institutions and different disciplines have been trained in evidence-based research as CADENZA Fellows. Each fellow partnered with NGOs and developed a project that the program had the potential to be taken up as part of the regular community services.

3.5 Achievements and Impacts

The CADENZA Project has gone beyond just figures and statistics collected from different projects and activities and have made important achievements with significant impact on the society. This section describes CADENZA main achievements and its impact in each of its components:

3.5.1 *Public education*

Through a series of public education programs, CADENZA has raised the awareness of the positive aging messages to majority of Hong Kong people. Moreover, CADENZA has published a series of reports collecting data on well-being and implications of the aging population on burden of common chronic diseases of Hong Kong elders. These reports are made available to the public and provide for the first time in Hong Kong which informs on health and social policies with respect to cost of care, service needs in hospitals and community, as well as long term care.

3.5.2 *Training*

CADENZA has enhanced the knowledge and skills in gerontology amongst different levels of professionals and front-line workers involved in elderly work as well as family carers and the general public. Through a series of training activities, over 13,000 people have been trained, including nurses, social workers, occupational therapists, physiotherapists and management executives. Feedback from the training programs indicated that participants found them very useful, not only in terms of skills, but also in the way they view and treat the people they serve.

3.5.3 *Community projects*

CADENZA has conducted a serious of community projects that enable collaborative NGOs to try out new care models to meet identified needs and to fill service gaps. Various service delivery models piloted and evaluated by the CADENZA project have also been integrated into the Hospital Authority services: hospital discharge support program in partnership with

NGOs; chronic disease self-management program; hospital referrals to user pays services — maximizing all community support in a flexible way for users; and end-of-life care training developed in Shatin Hospital to be diffused to residential care homes for the elderly; all in partnership with all service providers involved in care of the elderly. All these activities are in line with the recently developed Elder Care Strategy of the Hospital Authority, emphasizing the importance of Primary Care, as well as End-Of-Life Care. In addition, the concept of the CADENZA Hub has also been taken up by Hong Kong Housing Society in their development of elder housing.

3.5.4 *Leadership training*

CADENZA has also made a significant contribution to leadership training in the area of elderly care through its Fellowship training program. Since 2007, 30 faculty members from various tertiary institutions and different disciplines have been trained in evidence-based research. They have developed various community services to meet older people's needs. Some of the Fellows projects such as insomnia groups in the Hub and the post-retirement support and bereavement counseling are being introduced into the community as part of services.

3.6 Future Plans

From 2010 onwards, CADENZA will partner with Hong Kong Council of Social Service to launch a territory-wide public education program on Age-Friendly City (AFC) to raise public awareness of the AFC concept and creating an elderly-friendly environment in Hong Kong. CADENZA will also collaborate with Jockey Club Center for Positive Aging to launch a series of public education events and activities to promote brain health and to prevent dementia. CADENZA will continue the online training program and accompanying workshops and clinical attachments to provide multi-level education and training to different levels of professionals and front-line workers involved in elderly work as well as family carers and the general public. CADENZA will also involve different partners and stakeholders (such as NGOs and Social Welfare Department) to develop community projects and pioneer new service models to provide support for formal, informal carers and hidden elderly. A major effort will also be directed at the CADENZA Hub, as it has just started operation. CADENZA will review existing Hub training courses and strengthen their programs on dementia care, residential home care and disease prevention and management. Last but not the least, CADENZA will continue to arrange presentation of completed projects and promote uptake of programs in regular community services offered by NGOs regarding the leadership training component.

3.7 Conclusion

With aging, there are inevitable physical and mental changes. These changes must be dealt with in a positive way not only by individuals, but also by society. Since 2006, CADENZA has engaged partners from different organizations, institutions and professions to initiate positive changes towards an age-friendly Hong Kong through professional education, training, raising public awareness and supporting community demonstration projects, underpinned by evidence-based practice. A series of research activities has been carried out to gather data and evidence to provide rationale for public education programs, community projects and training program. Through survey and group discussions, knowledge gaps and misconceptions about aging were determined and service needs were identified. Results of the research activities and service evaluation have been disseminated through 18-district public education programs, TV series, press conferences, symposia as well as media interviews and articles. These public education activities as well as the development of community projects and training program revolved around the themes of active aging, empowerment, as well as health and social service interface. Following on what have been achieved; CADENZA will continue to initiate positive changes towards an age-friendly Hong Kong. It is hoped that these changes will stimulate others, including government and various NGOs, focusing on the needs of the elderly throughout Hong Kong and to benefit various organizations involved in caring of the elderly, different levels of health and social care professionals as well as people of all ages from all walks of life. This helps create an age-friendly environment in Hong Kong which fosters positive community attitude towards aging and improves the quality of care and quality of life of older people.

References

2007. http://wwwcenstatdgovhk/products_and_services/products/publications/statistical_report/population_and_vital_events/index_cd_B112001503_dt_detailjsp.

Census and Statistics Department of Hong Kong Special Administrative Region. Hong Kong population projections 2007–2036.

Johri, M., Beland, F. and Bergman, H. (2003) International experiments in integrated care for the elderly: a synthesis of the evidence. *Int. J. Geriatr. Psychiatry* **18**, 222–235.

Chapter 4

Longevity, Life Satisfaction, Money and Aging

David Schnaiter

Abstract

The demographic change, its origins and its challenges for politics and medicine, is one of the most important topics in actual health-related research. Regrettably most of this research neglects non-clinical aspects and is not willing to consider *soft facts* like self-referenced well-being or perceived health. Bringing together actual health-related findings from different disciplines working in life satisfaction research, an introduction and overview on the current state of discussion with strong focus on the elderly shall be provided — it aims to show that life satisfaction is one of the most decisive factors for healthy aging and longevity.

Core aspects are the amazing relationship between well-being, self-referenced health and classical parameters like life expectancy, the question on the impact of money and the satisfaction paradox of the old.

Keywords: Aging; Life Satisfaction; Perceived Health; Determinants; New Public Health; Research Synthesis.

4.1 The Demographic Shift and the Search for its Reasons

The demographic shift and the changes and challenges our societies are facing are greatly stressed topics in recent years. To identify these challenges for politics *and* for medicine, life expectancy is still one of the most important parameters for the evaluation of health politics and strategies — even though knowledge gaps and missing strategic orientation are getting more and more obvious, especially in the so-called developed world.

When looking at these economically developed countries a rather continuous progress of life expectancy gains during the last 150 years is to be stated, despite cohort effects like industrialization, famine episodes, World Wars I and II, etc. Currently life expectancy at birth rises about three months a year or three hours a day in these countries. The United Nations had to alter their estimates three times within the last 20 years (compare with e.g. Kirkwood, 2008). The estimates were wrong because the basis for the calculations was wrong. We are facing a phenomenon hardly anybody is talking about yet: Until the late 1960s the rapidly declining early- and midlife mortality caused the major part of life expectancy gains in the economically developed world (the main reasons for these gains are hygiene, housing, food, education, sanitation, vaccines, antibiotics, etc.). Since the beginning 1970s up to now early- and midlife mortality remained quite stable and late-life mortality declines are raising the overall life expectancy. This time the identifiable causes were strongly related to medicare and health care technologies and systems. But survival rates and long term treatment are explaining only a part of the life expectancy gains … a conclusive explanation for the reductions in late-life mortality is missing — certainly it is not due to medicine alone!

Our next thought would be immediately: general living circumstances related to income and money. On most Preston-curves we can observe a direct relation between money (GDP per capita) and life expectancy up to a point where basic primary needs can be sufficiently fulfilled. This would actually be between US$3 and about US$5 in power parity terms per head and year. After this borderline the automatism of the relation starts fading and when arriving at the higher incomes it is mostly lost. Wilkinson and Pickett (2009) state: There is a "ceasing relation above US$25 GDP/c".

UNDP's harshly criticized Human Life Development Index HDI (still) depends by two-thirds on life expectancy at birth and GDP per capita in purchase power parity terms, but both parameters are not very useful any more for strategic health policy planning and public health oriented comparisons between economically developed countries. So the classical indicators of mortality, life expectancy, GDP, etc. remain important, but their significance is clearly limited and leads to a dead end — we have to consider necessary expansions.

4.2 Necessary Expansions

A major reason for the need for other parameters is that when talking about late life and medical care we have to consider the fact that the point of time of getting ill lies very often years before death. We have to deal with

- chronic diseases and handicaps;
- reduced mobility;
- need for care; and
- mental illnesses, etc.

It's the restrictions in a patient's quality of life that are posing the biggest challenges for (geriatric) medicine and health politics in the economically developed world. So, if we accept that quality of life and well-being are important factors in health assessments, we need appropriate ways of measuring it. The two basic approaches are: indexing objective living conditions through indicator-based data-comparisons between collectives, and asking for subjective perceptions by using self-references through a questionnaire. Study results issued within the last few years are extremely promising: Direct and highly significant correlations with classical medical factors (longevity, mortality, morbidity, lifestyle factors, suicide rate, healthy life expectancy, disability adjusted life years, burden of disease, etc.) but also with classical social scientific topics (politics, democracy level, participation, personal freedom, environment, economy, and so on) could be confirmed. In comparison life satisfaction research (respectively research on well-being/happiness — terms used unfortunately quite interchangeable in literature) shows the better results. In large studies, authors from all over the world are proving that life satisfaction is demonstrating to be maybe the most important pro-factor for health in general. E.g. Bjørnskov was able to demonstrate (data from World Value Survey) the bivariate association between life expectancy as classical parameter for health and the degree of satisfaction with life — and proved its strong correlation (0.52) and significance ($p < 0.01$) across the world (Bjϕrnskov, 2008). The life expectancy of happy individuals is seven to ten years higher than the one of rather unhappy people within the same countries — an outcome comparable to the well-accepted correlation between smoking and longevity (Veenhoven, 2008).

4.3 Money and Life Satisfaction

So what is it that makes us happy? If we have a glimpse on the geographic distribution of happy and unhappy societies around the globe we get to see an image that is not really surprising and that seems to indicate again that money is the crucial cause for happiness. But is it really the money? Money has been the most discussed topic in life satisfaction research, especially after Easterlin postulated his paradox in 1974 (Easterlin, 1974; Easterlin, 1995).

It is to say that without any doubt fundamental basic needs have to be fulfilled before it makes sense to evaluate happiness levels. Therefore raising the overall income and in this way the individual possibility of assuring ones own existence in financially underdeveloped countries is crucial. But looking e.g. at the US, we observe a rather constant level of satisfaction with life since World War II that is not merely depending on Gross National Product development (compare, e.g., Diener and Biswas-Diener, 2002; Diener and Seligman, 2001, and many others more). Nevertheless

Table 4.1. The currently most important data bases related to life satisfaction research (in alphabetical order).

CIA World Factbook
Eurobarometer
European Social Survey (ESS)
Gallup World Poll
Happy Planet Index
National surveys
OECD Factbook
Penn World Tables
UN Human Development Report
UNESCO
UNICEF index on child wellbeing
WHO health for all database
World Bank: World Development Report
World Data Base of Happiness
World Value Surveys

there is a fierce dispute on the impact of money on life satisfaction and happiness going on at the moment — with lots of political and economic outreach.

Fact is that when looking at the relationship between GDP per capita and life satisfaction, we can observe a similar phenomenon as with life expectancy and money, even if more deviation is to be stated. Again there is an obvious borderline: primary needs must be fulfilled and up to this point no gains in life satisfaction are to be made. As demonstrated by numerous studies the strong correlation between absolute income and happiness starts fading over time when passing by the threshold of extreme poverty and adding an extra (compare e.g., Pugno, 2009).

While criticized in its details, Easterlin's (Easterlin, 2001; 2006; 2009), Wilkinson's (Gardner *et al.*, 1994; Wilkinson and Pickett, 2007; Wilkinson and Pickett, 2006) and others' fundamental findings are a fact: Although remaining an important aspect, a constant and robust association between absolute income and happiness over time in *rich* countries is not given and remains inconsistent. Satisfaction with life seems to follow Maslow's hierarchy of needs (Maslow, 1943) and passes on to the next levels when primary physical needs are fulfilled. Obviously personal and social priorities change at this point. Lifestyle and other factors become more dominant. Money still remains a decisive factor but others gain more importance. Thus relative income hypothesis became a central happiness research object, showing the significance of relative deprivation, diverging income distribution, rising expectations and economic inequalities within societies and well-being (e.g, Alesina *et al.*, 2004; Binswanger, 2006; Caporale *et al.*, 2009; Karlsson *et al.*, 2010; O'Connell, 2004).

The great health relevance of income-associated social comparison was proven for abundant health indicators like overall mortality and life expectancy (Cristia, 2009; Kawachi and Kennedy, 1997; Mc Isaac and Wilkinson, 1997), CVD risk factors (ez-Roux *et al.*, 2000), mental illness (Pickett *et al.*, 2006), obesity (Pickett *et al.*, 2005), self-rated health (Lopez, 2004; Subramanian *et al.*, 2001), etc.

At this stage life satisfaction research and some of its major proponents dare to step on even thinner ice. Keely speaks of a hedonic treadmill the propensity to consume led us (Keely, 2005; Pugno, 2009). The "buying happiness problem" not only splits scientists but also has a strong ideological context. Sophisticated comments and arguments related to this topic show how profoundly important lifestyle defence and national cultures are.

4.4 Other Determinants of Life Satisfaction

Even though causality and interdependencies remain a rather unsolved question so far and there is still quite a lot of research is to be done, there are already more than a few hints on what determines our happiness. These factors besides money are currently being identified within numerous studies on life satisfaction from all scientific disciplines.

After a period of focusing a bit disproportionately on income-related happiness research, the search for other (co-)determinants seems to gain importance (again). Even though causality and interdependencies remain a rather unsolved question so far, it becomes more and more clear that our state of well-being and happiness depends on an interrelated network of external-systemic and individual determinants.

Individual happiness is, like hardly every health-related topic, strongly correlated with demographic factors, educational level, gender and diversity aspects (Arrindell and Veenhoven, 2002), religious affiliation (Mookerjee and Beron, 2005) and ethnicity (Oppenheimer, 2001). Working conditions (Pouwels *et al.*, 2008) and country economics (Peiró, 2006) are of special interest — and closely related to the decisive psychological factors (Rotter, 1990), social capital and support (Verme, 2009), sociocultural variables, environmental quality (Brereton *et al.*, 2008; Rehdanz and Maddison, 2005; Welsch, 2007), sustainability (Gowdy, 2005; Zidansek, 2007) and individual values.

4.5 Subjective Health and Aging

What is especially interesting when talking about the demographic shift and aging is the issue of *health status* as one of the most important determinants of satisfaction with life. But unfortunately objective health status is a very difficult variable as it does not always show generalizable results. Aging is inevitably affected by a steady objective health decline which harshly influences our well-being and quality of life. Within the past few

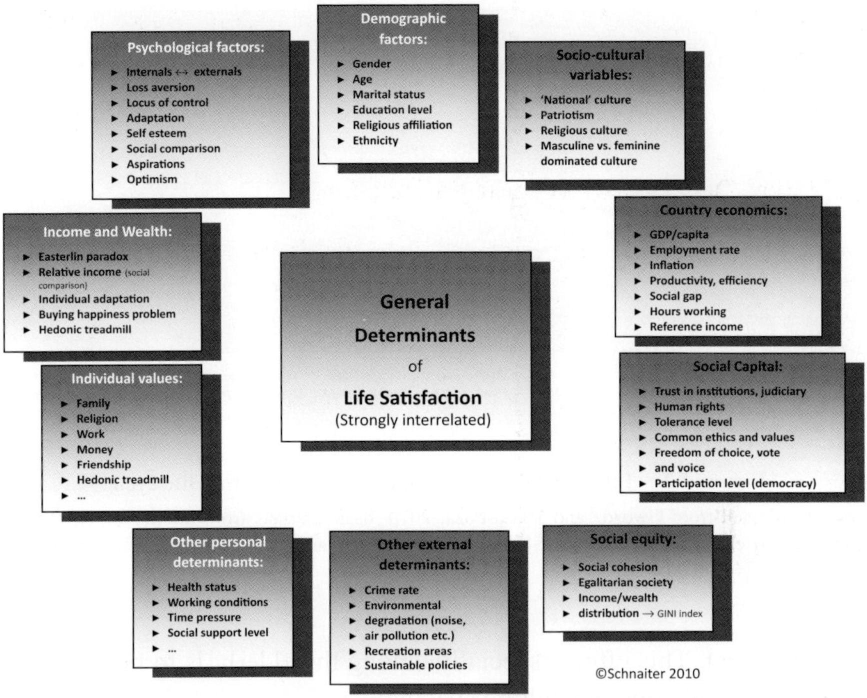

Figure 4.1. Overview on general determinants of life satisfaction.

years however, numerous studies were able to show that the classical parameters of clinical health status analysis have less to do with longevity, healthy aging, quality of life and happiness of the elderly as we all believed for quite a long time.

But the parameter subjective health status does and it shows amazing results! In fact it gets more and more obvious that self-referenced subjective health is a decisive parameter for healthy and happy aging *and* risen life expectancy. Among the many aspects influencing the relationship between health and well-being the effect of subjective health on life satisfaction and vice versa is significant in all specifications and therefore especially interesting.

Self-reported state of health influences well-being a lot more than the outcome of objective health parameters measured (compare e.g. Chen and Short, 2008; Gwozdz and Sousa-Poza, 2010; Smith *et al.*, 2002, and many

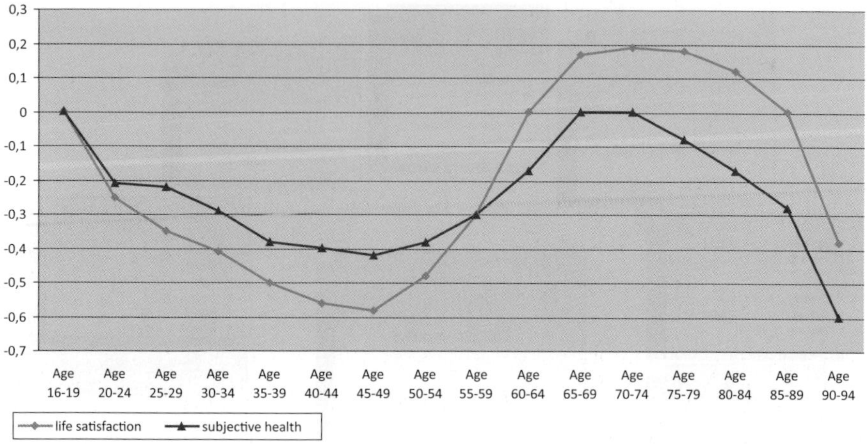

Figure 4.2. Life satisfaction and subjective health during life cycle.

Source: Adapted from Gwozdz and Sousa-Poza, 2010: basic datasets from the Survey on Health, Aging and Retirement in Europe (SHARE) and the German Socio-Economic Panel [GSOEP] 1994–2006, $n = 240.98$.

more studies). This effect especially among the elderly is to be observed around the world and not culture specific.

When looking at Fig. 4.2 we see at first sight that subjective health and life satisfaction do correlate very well. At second sight we notice the U-shaped form. After adolescence life satisfaction and subjective health are in constant decline until they reach their all-time low at the age of 45. Then both start zooming up until they reach their all-time peak at the age of 70 to 74. At this point subjective health and life satisfaction get caught up by objective health and a constant and harsh decline until death is inevitable (in older literature this dramatic decline is in most cases already reached at the age of 65). Thus, life satisfaction in oldest age is assumed to be inevitably and directly affected by (objective) health. But up to this point a rather surprising phenomenon is to be observed: The self-reported state of health influences well-being more than measured health parameters — until the oldest old.

Interpretations of this U-shaped correlation point to two major causes: cohort experiences (e.g. the World War II generation in Europe etc.), and adaptation effects (with age you cope better and better with your personal strengths and — even more importantly — weaknesses). Most studies so far made refer to such a robust U-shaped relationship between age and levels of life satisfaction in all cohorts until the oldest age (compare especially Blanchflower and Oswald, 2008; Easterlin, 2006).

4.6 The Satisfaction Paradox of the Old

Health is not a goal by itself, health is a potential enabling us to do things that are important to us. This is apparent in recent gerontological literature, showing that especially comparably *small burdens of disease* affecting mobility, social participation and interaction, personal freedom and independency define subjective health. First of all, visible impairment, hearing defects, loss of basic physical mobility, incontinency, etc., are decisive for the perceived health status and not the — from a medical point of view — more severe life-threatening diseases and risks. The objective health status of an elder person can be quite critical but nevertheless perceived health may be fairly good and life satisfaction in comparison to much younger people very high (a special case are mental illnesses, in particular dementia). This effect is called *satisfaction paradox of the old.*

The key function for subjective well-being is identified to be social participation and changing expectations at old age (for a very good description of this fact have, for example, a look at: Berg, *et al.*, 2006; 2009). Physical handicaps impeding social participation (immobility, sense impairments etc.) do limit to a very large extent the possibilities of social interaction, personal freedom and independency. At this point a vast difference between objective medical parameters and their understanding by medical experts and the reality of subjective well-being of a patient is to be stated. The strong and decisive interdependencies of life satisfaction, objective and perceived health are still not common sense in the life sciences. Maybe a re-orientation/adaptation of health sciences is necessary. From the satisfaction of physiological (primary) needs as determining factors of health in the economically developed countries to an increasing significance of non-biological factors: the psycho-social environment in all its diversity.

4.7 Conclusions

The WHO defines health as a "state of complete physical, mental and social well-being and not merely the absence of disease or infirmity" (WHO, 1948). Thus, health is already by definition associated with the individual state of well-being and the cited recent studies evidence the impact of life satisfaction on life expectancy and other most important classical health indicators. It's a mutually dependant cycle. Nevertheless life satisfaction research suffers from its affective origins and is still not considered as it should be in medical sciences. Especially when *happiness* gets assessed many scientists still close all doors (and ears). But happiness research and its output are underestimated — especially in medical sciences. This gets particularly obvious when looking at the strong interrelationships found between life satisfaction and life expectancy. Satisfaction-related health research is already playing a key-role in New Public Health and looking at the broad spectrum of interdependent determinants, health care professionals will have to accept shifting paradigms. Health promotion by encouraging individual life abilities and socio-economics through the improvement of social, political and environmental livabilities have the strongest impact on a population's overall health status and health behaviour, and not merely curative activities. Addressing finally whole populations and not only the ill is the mission to achieve rapprochements towards a "state of complete physical, mental and social well-being".

Satisfaction with life is the figurehead of health-empowered people, especially when getting older.

References

Alesina, A., Di Tella, R. and MacCulloch, R. (2004). Inequality and happiness: are Europeans and Americans different? *J. Public Econ.* **88**, 2009–2042.

Arrindell, W.A. and Veenhoven, R. (2002). Feminine values and happy life-expectancy in nations. *Pers. Indiv. Diff.* **33**, 803–813.

Berg, A.I., Hassing, L.B., McClearn, G.E. and Johansson, B. (2006). What matters for life satisfaction in the oldest-old? *Aging Ment. Health* **10**, 257–264.

Berg, A.I., Hoffman, L., Hassing, L.B., McClearn, G.E. and Johansson, B. (2009). What matters, and what matters most, for change in life satisfaction in the oldest-old? A study over 6 years among individuals 80+. *Aging Ment. Health* **13**, 191–201.

Binswanger, M. (2006). Why does income growth fail to make us happier? Searching for the treadmills behind the paradox of happiness. *J. Socio-Econ.* **35**, 366–381.

Bjornskov, C. (2008). Healthy and happy in Europe? On the association between happiness and life expectancy over time. *Soc. Sci. Med.* **66**, 1750–1759.

Blanchflower, D.G. and Oswald, A.J. (2008). Is well-being U-shaped over the life cycle? *Soc. Sci. Med.* **66**, 1733–1749.

Brereton, F., Clinch, J.P. and Ferreira, S. (2008). Happiness, geography and the environment. *Ecol. Econ.* **65,** 386–396.

Caporale, G.M., Georgellis, Y., Tsitsianis, N. and Yin, Y.P. (2009). Income and happiness across Europe: do reference values matter? *J. Econ. Psychol.* **30**, 42–51.

Chen, F. N. and Short, S.E. (2008). Household context and subjective well-being among the oldest old in China. *J. Fam. Issues* **29**, 1379–1403.

Cristia, J.P. (2009). Rising mortality and life expectancy differentials by lifetime earnings in the United States. *J. Health Econ.* **28**, 984–995.

Diener, E. and Biswas-Diener, R. (2002). Will money increase subjective well-being? *Soc. Indic. Res.* **57**, 119–169.

Diener, E. and Seligman, M.E.P. (2004). Beyond money. *Psychol. Sci. Public Interest* **5**, 1–31.

Easterlin, R.A. (1974). Does economic growth improve the human lot? In: *Nations and Households in Economic Growth: Essays in Honour of Moses Abramovitz* (eds.) David, P.A. and Reder, M.W. New York Academic Press, New York, pp. 89–125.

Easterlin, R.A. (1995). Will raising the incomes of all increase the happiness of all? *J. Econ. Behav. Organ* **27**, 35–47.

Easterlin, R.A. (2001). Subjective well-being and economic analysis: a brief introduction. *J. Econ. Behav. Organ.* **45**, 225–226.

Easterlin, R.A. (2006). Life cycle happiness and its sources: intersections of psychology, economics, and demography. *J. Econ. Psychol.* **27**, 463–482.

Easterlin, R.A. (2009). Lost in transition: life satisfaction on the road to capitalism. *J. Econ. Behav. Organ.* **71**, 130–145.

ez-Roux, A.V., Link, B.G. and Northridge, M.E. (2000). A multilevel analysis of income inequality and cardiovascular disease risk factors. *Soc. Sci. Med.* **50**, 673–687.

Gardner, S., Farrer, M., Munro, J., St Leger, A.S. and Wilkinson, R. (1994). Inequalities and health. *Lancet* **343**, 537–538.

Gowdy, J. (2005). Toward a new welfare economics for sustainability. *Ecol. Econ.* **53**, 211–222.

Gwozdz, W. and Sousa-Poza, A. (2010). Aging, health and life satisfaction of the oldest old: an analysis for Germany. *Social Indic. Res.* **97**, 397–417.

Karlsson, M., Nilsson, T., Lyttkens, C.H. and Leeson, G. (2010). Income inequality and health: importance of a cross-country perspective. *Soc. Sci. Med.* **70**, 875–885.

Kawachi, I. and Kennedy, B.P. (1997). The relationship of income inequality to mortality: does the choice of indicator matter? *Soc. Sci. Med.* **45**, 1121–1127.

Keely, L.C. (2005). Why isn't growth making us happier? Utility on the hedonic treadmill. *J. Econ. Behav. Organ.* **57**, 333–355.

Kirkwood, T.B.L. (2008). A systematic look at an old problem. *Nature* **451**, 644–647.

Lopez, R. (2004). Income inequality and self-rated health in US metropolitan areas: a multi-level analysis. *Soc. Sci. Med.* **59**, 2409–2419.

Maslow, A.H. (1943). A theory of human motivation. *Psychol. Rev.* **50**, 370–396.

McIsaac, S.J. and Wilkinson, R.G. (1997). Income distribution and cause-specific mortality. *Eur. J. Public Health* **7**, 45–53.

Mookerjee, R. and Beron, K. (2005). Gender, religion and happiness. *J. Socio-Econ.* **34**, 674–685.

O'Connell, M. (2004). Fairly satisfied: economic equality, wealth and satisfaction. *J. Econ. Psychol.* **25**, 297–305.

Oppenheimer, V.K. (2001). Social demography: role of inequality and social differentiation. In: *International Encyclopedia of the Social and Behavioral Sciences* (eds.) Neil, J.S. and Paul, B.B. (eds.) Pergamon, Oxford, pp. 14270–14276.

Peiró, A. (2006). Happiness, satisfaction and socio-economic conditions: some international evidence. *J. Socio-Econ.* **35**, 348–365.

Pickett, K.E., Kelly, S., Brunner, E., Lobstein, T. and Wilkinson, R.G. (2005). Wider income gaps, wider waistbands? An ecological study of obesity and income inequality. *J. Epidemiol. Commun. H.* **59**, 670–674.

Pickett, K.E., James, O.W. and Wilkinson, R.G. (2006). Income inequality and the prevalence of mental illness: a preliminary international analysis. *J. Epidemiol. Commun. H.* **60**, 646–647.

Pouwels, B., Siegers, J. and Vlasblom, J.D. (2008). Income, working hours, and happiness. *Econ. Lett.* **99**, 72–74.

Pugno, M. (2009). The Easterlin paradox and the decline of social capital: an integrated explanation. *J. Socio-Econ.* **38**, 590–600.

Rehdanz, K. and Maddison, D. (2005). Climate and happiness. *Ecol. Econ.* **52**, 111–125.

Rotter, J.B. (1990). Internal versus external control of reinforcement: a case history of a variable. *Am. Psychol.* **45**, 489–493.

Smith, J., Borchelt, M., Maier, H. and Jopp, D. (2002). Health and well-being in the young old and oldest old. *J. Soc. Issues* **58**, 715–732.

Subramanian, S.V., Kawachi, I. and Kennedy, B.P. (2001). Does the state you live in make a difference? Multilevel analysis of self-rated health in the US. *Soc. Sci. Med.* **53**, 9–19.

Veenhoven, R. (2008). Healthy happiness: effects of happiness on physical health and the consequences for preventive health care. *J. Happiness Stud.* **9**, 449–469.

Verme, P. (2009). Happiness, freedom and control. *J. Econ. Behav. Organ.* **71**, 146–161.

Welsch, H. (2007). Environmental welfare analysis: a life satisfaction approach. *Ecol. Econ.* **62**, 544–551.

WHO definition of health (1948). Preamble to the Constitution of the World Health Organization, International Health Conference, New York, 19–22 June, 1946; signed on 22 July 1946 by the representatives of 61 States (Official Records of the World Health Organization, No. 2, p. 100) and entered into force on 7 April 1948, 100. 7–4–1948.

Wilkinson, R.G. and Pickett, K.E. (2006). Income inequality and population health: a review and explanation of the evidence. *Soc. Sci. Med.* **62**, 1768–1784.

Wilkinson, R.G. and Pickett, K.E. (2007). The problems of relative deprivation: why some societies do better than others. *Soc. Sci. Med.* **65**, 1965–1978.

Wilkinson, R. and Pickett, K. (2009). *The Spirit Level: Why More Equal Societies Almost Always Do Better*. Allen Lane, UK.

Zidansek, A. (2007). Sustainable development and happiness in nations. *Energy* **32**, 891–897.

Chapter 5

Understanding Between Generations: A Practicable Way to Help Create a Society Fit for All Ages

Christa Erhart, Susanne Schinagl and Peter Erhart

Abstract

In 1999 the theme for the International Year of Older Persons was 'A Society for All Ages'. As a contribution and a practicable answer the Department of Geriatrics — Paracelsus Medical University Salzburg (Head HR Prim. Dr. Peter Erhart) presented the primary preventive teaching project 'One step towards old age'. We targeted all generations to participate in social commitments and lifelong learning. The first step involved the young generation.

The main element of this project is a three-hour adventure world "The Arena of Daily Living" located at the Department of Geriatrics. Based on a new scientific and didactic approach we started to raise awareness for an unacquainted period of life. The participants work with special devices designed to experience old age by imitation.

Our message is: 'Old age is not a handicap to man but man is a handicap to old age'. A short description of the workshop explains how to achieve key priorities like highlighting a positive view of aging, understanding the meaning of "WE" in a society, knowledge on the aging process in connection with environmental challenges, awareness of the stressful combination of physiological changes and circumstances that put older persons at risk.

In 2002 we extended the project to the next two generations. Modules have been fitted into university teaching, nursing schools and academies. Special attention is given to geragogics and a cross-generation dialog. Lectures, meetings and trainings support independent living. Our homepage (www.zgb.at) serves as a platform for all generations.

Up till today, about 12,000 participants have attended our project.

Illustration and didactic support: Christian Tschepp

Keywords: Understanding between Generations; International Year of Older Persons; Second World Assembly on Aging; Lifelong Learning; Primary Preventive Teaching Project; Age Simulation; Arena of Daily Living; Handicap-Friendly Environment; Images of Old Age; Cross-Generational Dialog; Generation Interpreter.

Quality of life in the elderly is highly dependent on intergenerational understanding. This positive interchange of information, thoughts and opinions encounters bio-psycho-social barriers and demands life skills from all involved parties.

Extrinsic factors, in particular inadequate physical surroundings and a low awareness of this period of life, contribute a considerable part to the individual aging process. The lack of understanding of older persons, often due to a lack of knowledge and awareness, can contribute to a loss of independence, illness and eventually to a growing need of special care or even social marginalization amongst the aged. This calls for a concerted responsibility and learning principles for young and old including attitude, knowledge and skills. We need all generations to participate in social commitments and lifelong learning. Only by getting to know each other mutually, and by learning to identify age-related changes and the resulting problems, could understanding between generations be imagined.

In 1999 the theme for the International Year of Older Persons was "A Society for All Ages". The aim of that year was to promote awareness for the issue of aging in our society. Researchers, politicians, and practitioners were called on to take the initiative in ensuring the integration of old people into all sectors of society and in creating opportunities integral to all stages of life.

As a contribution and a practicable answer we presented the primary preventive teaching project "One Step towards Old Age" (Fig. 5.1).

The first step involved the young generation. There we took a new approach based on the idea that our children and teenagers are the architects of tomorrow's world. Soon it will be their responsibility to create an environment, which ensures security and quality of life for everybody — a world without barriers and obstacles, with products designed for young and old.

Based on a completely new scientific and didactic approach we started to raise awareness for what "WE" means in a society as early as possible. This aim is not attained by wagging one's finger, but with educationally focused fun and games. Step by step we included all generations to

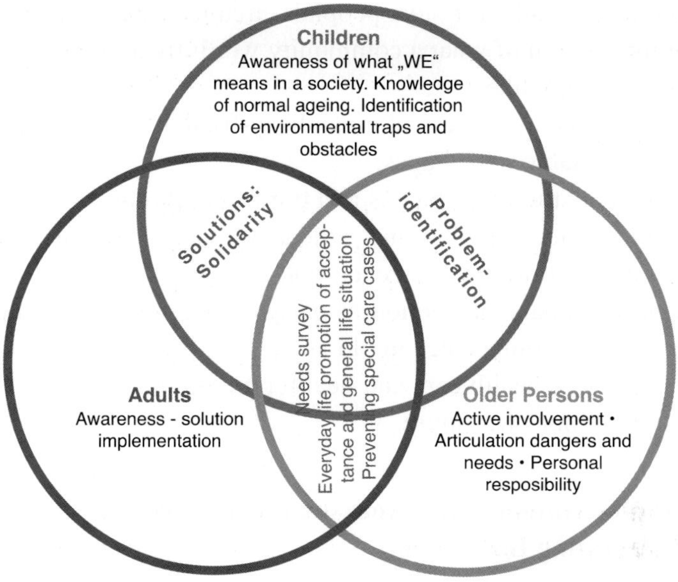

Figure 5.1. All three generations contribute to healthy aging and a sense of security in old age.

participate in our scheme. The main element of this project is a three-hour adventure world "The Arena of Daily Living" located at the Department of Geriatrics/Paracelsus Medical University Salzburg. The children work with special devices designed to experience old age by imitation. Together we develop visions of a future worthwhile for all ages. The message behind our approach is: "Aging is normal' and 'Old age is not a handicap to man but man is a handicap to old age". We have a team of qualified partners assisting us with meeting the special needs. For this reason, we cooperate closely with the International Academy of Sciences in Innsbruck.

In 2001 the staff, administration and financially related investments were too high for a hospital and we founded the "Zentrum für Generationen und Barrierefreiheit — ZGB" (Centre for Generations and Accessibility). From this point on the organization worked independently remaining however in close cooperation with the Department of Geriatrics.

The project is launched with the aim of:

- contributing to a more positive image of old age;
- emphasising aging as an asset;

- promoting empathy for older people's circumstances already in youth;
- creating a vision of what a community worth living in at all stages of life should look like;
- developing the awareness of a handicap-friendly environment and of products suitable for all ages;
- pointing out stumbling-blocks and traps in everyday life;
- improving understanding and solidarity among all generations and have a part in bridging the generation gap;
- providing primary prevention as early as possible to maintain independence and competence in old age;
- contributing to health care and health promotion; and
- investing in our own future.

5.1 Short Description of the Workshop with Children and Operating Instruction

The workshop is addressed to entire classes, their teachers and interested parents.

In a three-hour obstacle course adapted to the needs of ten-year-olds everyday obstacles for older people are experienced realistically.

5.1.1 *Activity room 1: Classroom*

Five life-size role models made of wood guide through the activity rooms (Fig. 5.2). At a press of a button the figures raise typical children's questions

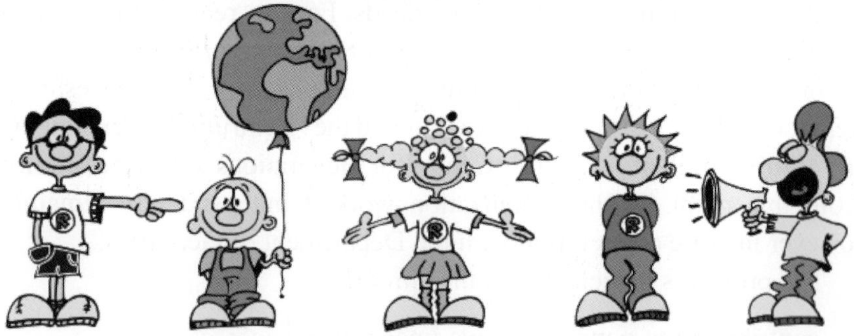

Figure 5.2. Role models.

and issues. Each of the characters is used as a key figure and a base for sustainability for the special issue that was discussed in the connecting activity room and reappears in our newsletter, "Makes Sense" children book, and teaching materials and on our internet platform. We worked out accurately defined goals for the individual rooms hidden in "evaluation stories". The participants meet in the "classroom". Daniel, the professor — role model for tricky questions, learning, and knowledge — tells the first evaluation story.

The key priorities of this room are: attitude, awareness, highlighting positive images of age, and understanding the meaning of "WE" in a society. We welcome the class and divide it into small groups with their own group instructor. As conceptions and images of old age are determined early in life we implemented a special research on this subject. It is a key priority and an integral aspect of the workshops to promote images highlighting a positive view of aging; thereby misleading and negative stereotypes are eradicated.

After having introduced ourselves, we ask the key questions: "what do you think when you hear the terms old man, old woman, aging, to be old?" The answers are read to the children and discussed. Soon we realized a predominated ill-balanced sad picture of weakness, and pupils did not find positive aspects of aging with which they could identify in any way. Table 5.1 shows the result of an interim evaluation in 2005.

The basic questions were how to deal with this image, and how to fight the underlying worry? Let us put forth a piece of advice: Give these old people faces, names and feelings, and put them in everyday situations. Ask about personal experiences. For this purpose we created a "Generation Circle" (Fig. 5.3).

The pictures show different situations and associated feelings got matched with the generations. In place we gain the "Eureka Effect". Children realize that needs and feelings remain the same over the different periods of life, and understand the importance of satisfying basic needs.

Table 5.1. Image of old age in 10–15 year old pupils, n. 1111–1291 answers.

Positive	Neutral	Negative
2%	15%	83%

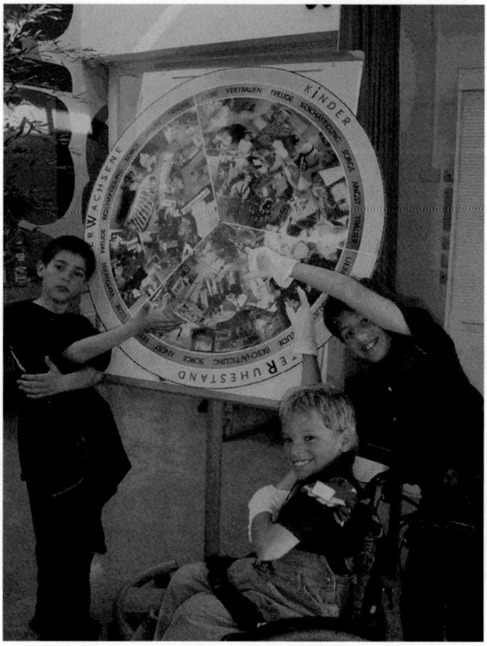

Figure. 5.3. Generation circle.

Diligently and well motivated they follow the instructions and try attentively to trace problems that could endanger older people. The foundations of the "WE" in a society for all ages are laid.

A further key priority is to communicate important physiological changes in connection with environmental challenges.

At that point we start our trip through time. First we explain tactile perception and the age-related changes. Equipped with special gloves, small differences at a special tactile board as well as the different euro coins can no longer be perceived. The physiological loss of receptors can be applied to the explanation of extremity position sense as well (Fig. 5.4). Children grasp the complex relationships in keeping balance and security. They learn that older persons are more likely to get stressed and need more time to perform to tap their full potential.

Next we deal with the sense of vision. The kids learn how the eye works and how to protect it optimally. With especially developed glasses we simulate some common age-related changes like the dry eye syndrome,

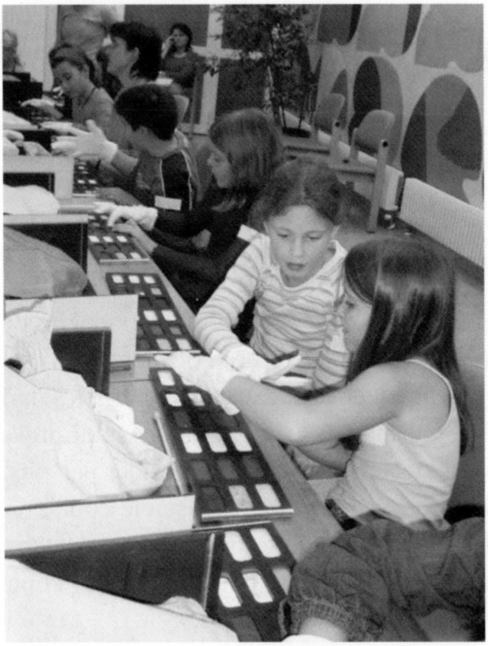

Figure 5.4. Classroom.

the physiological loss of light sensitivity and opacity, and yellowing of the lens. The loss of dynamic acuity is explained and experienced with different magnifiers.

Next, we talk about structural and functional changes of the ear, the best prevention starting already in youth and the upcoming problems in speech understanding, directional hearing and background noise. We insert some strategies like demonstrating the importance of the eye contact that builds a bridge for words and emotions. Moreover we point to babble of voices and stress a clear and slow verbal communication with older persons.

Finally, the class is subjected to a small stress test. Half of the pupils have to cope in a peaceful and friendly environment, the other half under stressful conditions. Usually the latter group reacts negatively affected and shows a much poorer result.

With such a basic knowledge and additionally handicapped with bandages, small weights, and a special waistcoat, the participants grow to

85 years of age. They are called on to detect stumbling blocks and traps in the different activity rooms and to report results and solutions at the final conference. A common goal for the different activity rooms is to make sure that children understood the theoretical lesson and deepening of learned communication strategies.

5.1.2 *Activity room 2: Outdoor activities*

Evaluation story: Great-grandma and the role model Frederic visit the doctor's surgery. A risky adventure for both of them.

Key priorities: Knowledge on gate-characteristics in old age, realizing the principle of "small matter — great effect", fall prevention, and what "mind the step" and "watch out!" mean for older persons.

Children pass through an ordinary obstacle course in a dimly lit corridor and a reach a staircase. There they mark dark steps with differently coloured glue strips and discover the importance of contrasts. Afterwards they discuss low cost solutions (Fig. 5.5).

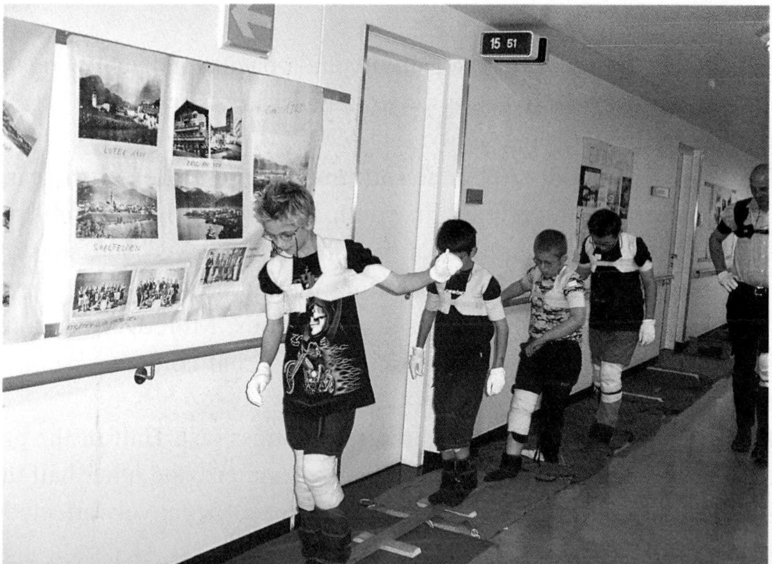

Figure 5.5. Outdoor activities.

5.1.3 *Activity room 3: Daily living*

Evaluation story: Shopping with grandma and how the role-model Chrissie can help with that difficult job.

Key priorities: Type faces, expiring data, where to put them and how to make them easy to read, usability.

Children make purchases, read hard to decipher bills, look for well-concealed expiring data, test different locks, fasteners and modern electronics and discuss low cost solutions (Fig. 5.6).

5.1.4 *Activity room 4: Hearing and mishearing*

Evaluation story: The role model Ben asks why he was perceived as cheeky and why an old lady felt offended by him.

Key priorities: The focus is directed not only on audibility but also on politeness and the specific language and neologisms that may involuntarily offend others (Fig. 5.7). (There we gained an important input for the book entitled "Oida a Generation Interpreter".)

Kids listen with headsets to situations especially adapted to the hearing capacity of old age and notice that background noise extinguishes the

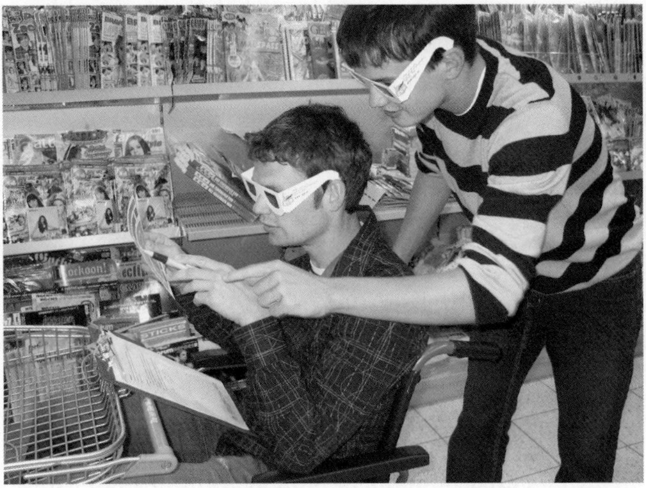

Figure 5.6. Daily living.

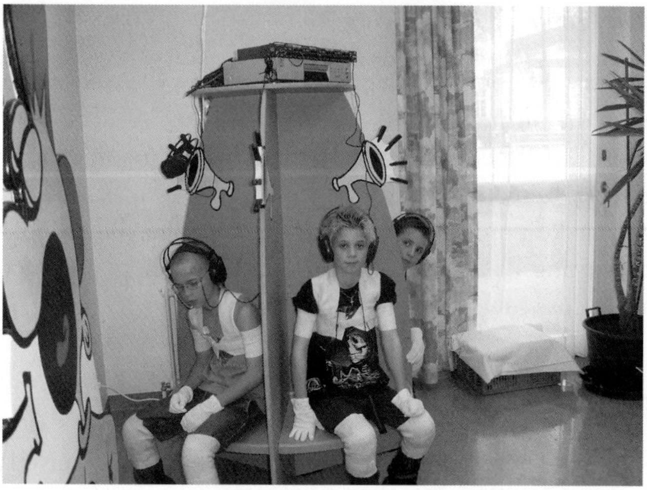

Figure 5.7. Listening.

spoken information. The concrete examples had been cut in a professional recording studio.

5.1.5 *Activity room 5: Public transport*

Evaluation story: After a long day at school Bine is tired and angry about a poor mark. She asks why she should leave her seat to an older man.

Key priorities: Awareness of the stressful combination of different physiological changes and circumstances that put older persons at risk. Discussion on older people's behavior patterns.

Standing on a shaky platform at our lifelike bus stop, children experience the task: holding a cane in one hand and a shopping bag in the other hand, getting on the bus, digging the ticket out of the burse stamping, maintaining balance and getting out of the bus as a challenge. Kids understand now, that unfriendliness is often a stress-governed reaction to fear of falling, instability and loss of balance (Fig. 5.8).

5.1.6 *Activity room 6: Children conference*

Empowered as detectives and the architects of tomorrow's world, the different groups are gathering at a flip chart and recording their findings and

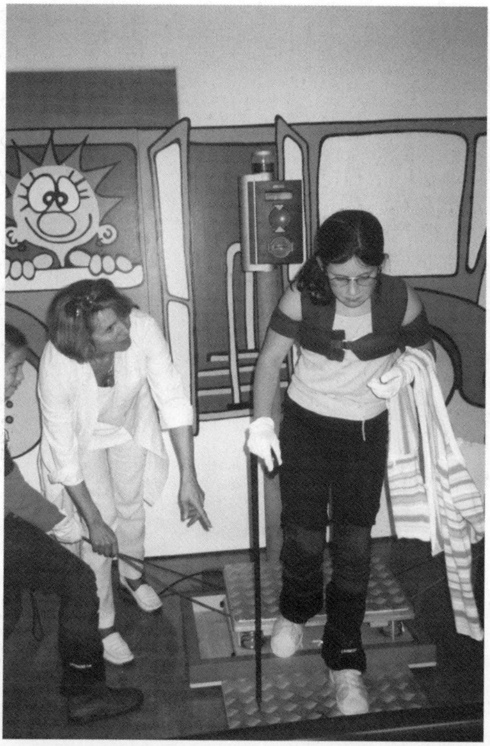

Figure 5.8. Public transport.

ideas in writing or drawing (Fig. 5.9). It is impressive to see the enthusiasm of the kids collaborating together and endearingly putting their requests and proposals. Data are extracted and validated by the different evaluation stories.

Sustainability:

(1) The textbook for children "Das macht Sinn" ("Makes sense"), subtitled "A book about our five senses", comprises adventure, games, experiments and background information on aging (Fig. 5.10). In 2001 three thousand books financed by a charity action had been distributed in Salzburg in all elementary schools at no cost to be used for teaching the subject of aging.
(2) Our Homepage (www.zgb.at) is a platform for all generations. Newsletters on the basis of competitions, experiments and thrilling

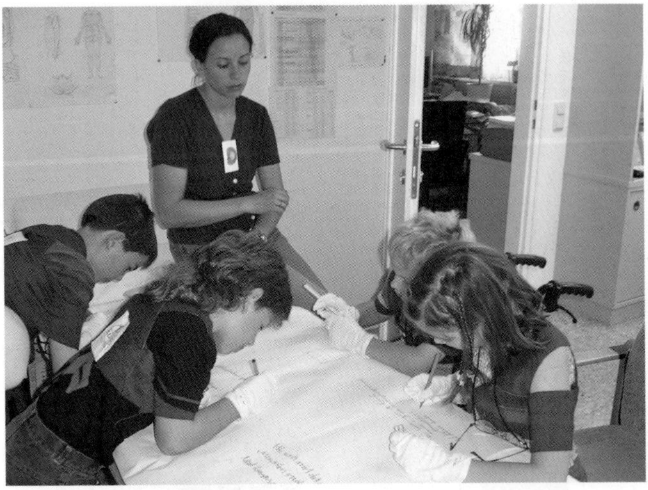

Figure 5.9. Conference.

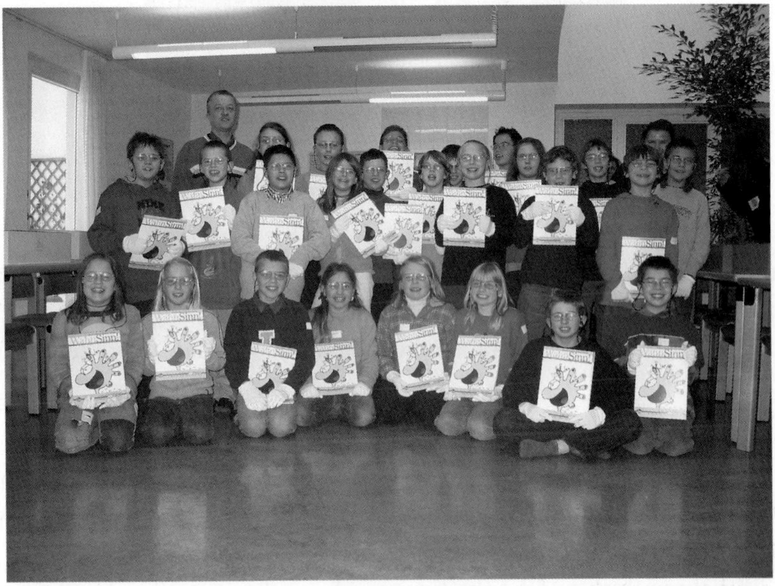

Figure 5.10. The textbook "Das macht Sinn".

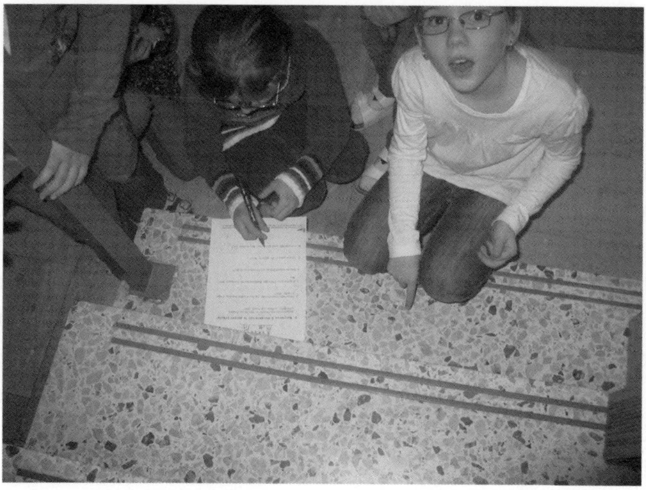

Figure 5.11. Detective day.

reports are published regularly for downloading with the aim to motivate children to work for a barrier-free environment. In our kids-corner, children find help in learning in alphabetic order. Additionally we have a didactical service providing teaching resources on special subjects.

(3) ZGB is engaged in Children University and regularly organized "Detective Days" (Fig. 5.11).

To work with children means to work for the future. Already, problems exist, and it is in all of our interest to solve them as quickly as possible. The maxim of physician's responsibility: "*Primum non Nocere*" must be applied in the context with the physical environment.

Strengthened in our resolve by the International Plan on Action adopted at the "Second World Assembly on Aging in Madrid 2002", we extended the scope of research to the next two generations and participated in the implementation.

The three priority directions respond to the opportunities and challenges of aging in the 21st century:

(1) older persons and development;
(2) advancing health and well-being into old age; and
(3) ensuring enabling and supportive environments,

Many recommendations for action and goals are in-line with the ideas and aims that we share in our three-generation project. Decades of clinical experience have sharpened our awareness of the cardinal problems of older persons. Measures to strengthen autonomy and self-determination in the elderly are the best assets to positive aging. The realization of these goals requires comprehensive intergenerational understanding, a positive image of old age and lifelong learning. To design products, provide services and to shape the environment frequently is the preserve of adults. Working people are hardly familiar with the shortcomings resulting from the physiological aging process. It is small wonder that there are wrongly designed products as well as failed adaptations of the environment. The issue of aging is still an educational blind spot. Active gerontology is requested.

As early as 1985 Bergener argued: "Taking gerontology as a model, a decisive alteration could and should take place to end the tyranny of a synthetic heuristic which predominates in all thinking throughout our occidental civilization. I am convinced that the clarification of gerontology's inner legitimacy depends very much on whether this change in our way of thinking really can be achieved. Otherwise gerontology may come to be regarded as a short-lived, pseudo-scientific fire fueled by fashionable words and phrases."

Whoever has put himself into someone else's shoes experiencing the other's physical reality, thinks and plans differently. Consequently, the adaptable simulation arena appropriate to instruct various occupational groups and the interested party is at the centre of presentation. A theoretical section dealing with the physiological changes in old age and with barrier-avoidance is adapted to the participants and their occupational interests. At the same time, corresponding written information material is supplied.

Modules have been introduced into university teaching, nursing schools and academies; theses on adequate shop design and product development have been supervised. Apart from advice, we provide product and service evaluation to help analyze criteria concerning user-friendliness and barrier avoidance; we also test younger and older individuals for the same purpose.

Special attention is paid to the work with older persons.

To grasp problems, we offer a helpline called "Trouble in everyday life". We point at the issue of falling, stress conduct and mobility. We aim at improving self-determination, self-image and preventive thinking. Along with handouts and brochures we developed a series of 22 gerontological lectures to be held at various institutions.

Promotion of an enabling environment for social development was one of the central objectives agreed upon at the World Summit for Social Development. Apart from good housing and an adapted environment, transportation is a growing concern. It is a fact that as people age they rely more heavily on appropriate public transport. Even to this issue, actions have been elaborated.

We arrange Mobility days and a "Bus training for Senior Citizens" in close cooperation with the public transport operator of our city. Finally we were partners in the AENEAS — EU Project. (Attaining Energy-Efficient Mobility in an Aging Society).

Our ambition is not only to create empathy for older persons but vice versa too.

An old saying goes, "People resemble their times more than they resemble their parents". There is much truth in it and characterizes our fast moving time. Consequently the generation of older people is called on to deal with the problems of the young.

To facilitate cross-generational dialog we organize meetings like: "Bring Generations together to Cook", and are partners of "Villages for Generations" and "Barrier-free Communities". In order to avoid language barriers, together with partners we published a book entitled "Oida! Der Generationen Dolmetscher" ("Oida the Generation Interpreter"), that shows how language has changed from generation to generation.

Until today about 12,000 participants have attended our project.

In the last few years the project received subsidisation from municipal, regional and national governmental sources. Unfortunately, in June 2010, parts of the project fell victim to the "global" financial crisis.

Hence, as soon as the schools closed for the summer we were forced to cease the provision of a number of core activities. Nevertheless with this approach we hope to have noticeably counteracted the environmental caused problems of older persons and disabled people and contributed to a better understanding between generations.

References

Arge Miteinander Reden, Hrsg. (2010) *Oida; Der Generationendolmetscher*. Verlag Anton Pustet.

Bergener, M. (1985) Introduction gerontology — between opportunity and reality. In: *Thresholds in Aging. The 1984 Sandoz Lectures in Gerontology* (eds.) Bergener, M., Ermini, M. and Stahelin, H.B. Academic Press Inc., London, pp. xiii–xix.

Erhart S. and Tschepp C. (2004) *Das macht Sinn, Das Erlebnis-Lern-Spiel-Buch über deine 5 Sinne und wie sie sich im Alter Verändern*. Verlag Junfermann, Stuttgart.

Erhart, C., Schinagl, S and Erhart, P. (2005) Umweltbedingte Gefährdungen der Lebensqualität im Alter. In: *Lebensqualität im Alter* (eds.) Likar, R., Bernatzky, G., Pipam, W., Janig, H. and Sadiak, A. Springer Verlag Hrsg, pp. 291–306.

United Nations (2002) Report of the Second World Assembly on Ageing, Madrid, 8–12 April 2002.

Chapter 6

The Life as a Struggle for Immortality: History of Ideas in Russian Gerontology (With Immunoneuroendocrine Bias)

Leonid P. Churilov and Yury I. Stroev

Abstract

The article is a review of ideas in Russian gerontology and geriatrics for 250 years. Most prominent concepts and figures in medical, biological and philosophical aspects of aging studies are shown, with accents made on immunoneuroendocrine mechanisms of senescence. The author's own studies, with reference to autoimmune thyroiditis, inherited disorders of connective tissue and accelerated aging are briefly characterized.

Keywords: Aging; Autoimmunity; Geriatrics; Gerontology; Immunoneuroendocrine Interactions; Russia; Thyroid Gland.

"Our strong desire to live is in contradiction with the diseases of senility and with the shortness of life. This is the greatest disharmony of the human nature"
Il'ya Mechnikov, On the Disharmonies of the Human Nature, 1904

The imperfection of human nature is manifested in mortality and senescence of a human being. The idea of eternal youth or attempts of rejuvenation were inherent to antique cultures from very old times. Perhaps, the earliest known system of hygienic measures for life prolongation, like low caloric diets and moderate hypoxic conditions of mountain walking, existed in practice of Daoism in ancient China of IV century B.C. (Gruman, 1966). But the Russian nation is very young: it has been ethnically entirely constituted only to late XIV century A.D. (Gumilev, 1990); that's why gerontological ideas only arose much later in Russian culture. In folk tales and medieval epos of Russians (Tolstoy, 1985), one can meet a hero named Ivan Tsarevich, the Tsar's junior son, sent by his father to remote country in seek for "the apples of rejuvenation". On the way Ivan got into many risky adventures and even was killed by enemies, but a kind magician (or the sorceress Baba Yaga) resurrected him with the help of "dead water" (that heals the wounds) and then "live water" (that puts life back into the body). Both dead and live waters were brought to magician in the beak of a wise crow. Interestingly, modern science appreciates the apples as a source of antioxidants, able to retard aging. Moreover, it confirms that in the course of any inflammation the production of cadaverine, putrescine and other polyamines of necrobiotic cells increases ("dead water"), which precedes the regeneration and is essential for anti-inflammatory and proliferative effects of wound healing (Zaichik and Churilov, 2008). The first mention of longevity problems in Russia ever occurred in authored texts belongs to Captain Jacques Margeret (ca. 1565–1619), who was employed to tsar Boris Godunov. This French mercenary in Russian service wrote in his book titled "Estate de l'Empire de Russie et de Grand Duché de Moscovie", dated 1606: "Many Russians live until 90–100 and 120 years and face illnesses only in an old age. Thus, nobody accepts medicines with the exception of the tsar and top noblemen". We do not know any professional Russian naturalists before the end of 17th century, but even among first Russian scientists of later period we can find deep interest in demography and studies of aging. The titanic figure of first Russian polymath Mikhailo Vasil'evich Lomonosov (1711–1765) stands there (see Fig. 6.1), with his contribution into all areas of knowledge — from physics to poetry. Lomonosov was a founder of Russian demography with his memo: "On the protection and proliferation of the people of Russia" (1761) addressed to Count Shuvalov, President of the Academy of Sciences, thus in 2011 we celebrated the 250th anniversary of domestic aging studies. The chapter contains a detailed analysis of the factors influencing mortality, birthrate and longevity of Russian population, with recommendations regarding social policy aimed at population growth (Lomonosov, 1950).

In 1754 *archiatros* (in fact, health minister of Empire in that period), Johann Bernhard von Fischer (1686–1772) published the first geriatric book in Russia ("*On Senility, its Degrees and Diseases*", republished in 1760), insisting that healthy senility is possible and putting the mark of

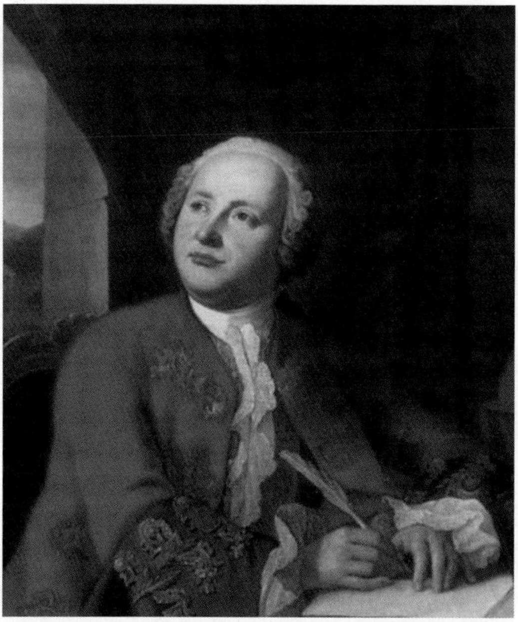

Figure 6.1. Originator of Russian Demography Mikhailo V. Lomonosov. Unknown painter of XVIII century. Oil/canvas. Lomonosov' s museum, Ust' Ruditsy, Arkhangelskaya region.

longevity to persons over 90 (Fischer, 1754). Because of cultural separation, the Western medieval fashion of occultism, hermetic philosophy and alchemy came to Russia very late and only spread among Russian aristocracy in late 18th century. Some of Russian occultists, all belonging to Masonic circles, equipped in Moscow and St. Petersburg alchemic laboratories and were involved in experiments with chemicals for achievement of eternal youth via "Philosophical Stone" or "Panacea" — the all-healing remedy.

Among them we shall mention in Moscow, Nicolay I. Novikov (1744–1818), and in St. Petersburg, Ivan P. Elagin (1725–1794), who kept an alchemic laboratory under one of the pavilions of his palace (Fig. 6.2) and in 1779, invited to his laboratory known European occultist and alchemist Giuseppe Balsamo (aka count Alessandro di Cagliostro, 1743–1795). Balsamo has demonstrated in Russia several alchemic experiments, propagating his "drug of transformation, in 40 days putting

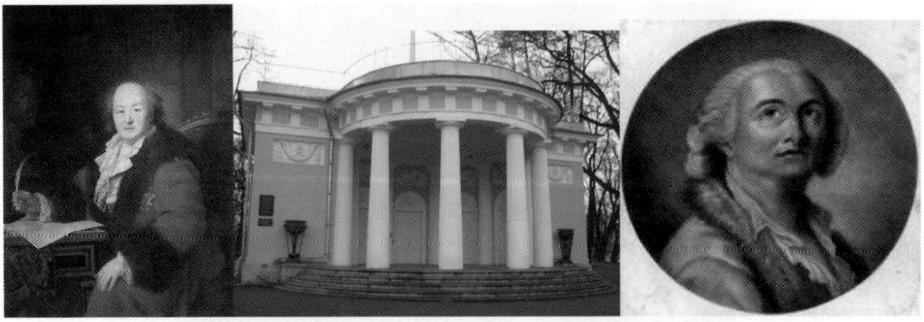

Figure 6.2. Count Ivan P. Elagin (by Jean-Louis Voille, oil/canvas, State Russian Museum, St. Petersburg) — *left*; Pavilion with Rotunda in his palace at St. Petersburg, under which alchemic laboratory was located; Giuseppe Balsamo, invited by Elagin and worked in Russia in 1779.

a person first in convulsions, than in deep sleeping and finally through teeth, skin and hair renewal — into rejuvenation". He even performed once a "resurrection" of a dead newborn son of another alchemist — Count Stroganov (later on it appeared that Balsamo simply changed the baby on the quiet) (Churilov and Shmeliov, 2008).

In 19th century, the founder of Genetics and Age Biology, German zoologist August Weismann (1860–1912), made many contributions to the science of aging (Fig. 6.3, left). Weismann (1881) formulated his understanding of aging as follows (Weismann, 1882), "The final reason, which determines lifetime, is the wear, to which the individuals undergo during their existence. Death seemed to me expedient, since the worn individuals for the species do not have a price and even they are harmful, taking space away from the best ones". According to the Weismann's ideas, the aging was elaborated evolutionarily during a transfer from the immortal unicellular to the mortal multicellular organisms, on the basis of so-called "retrogressive evolution mechanism", like other adaptations, deprived of the adaptive value and regressing into the rudiments (let say, eyesight in underground animals). Nature did not choose the pathway of improving the body's reactivity to the level of individual immortality achievement, because it proved to be evolutionarily cheaper to create "single-time case" for the immortal cells of germ line. Therefore "the soma", being imperfect, is worn out, which leads to a drop in the reproductive potential of cells (or according another Weismann's version, this potential is primarily

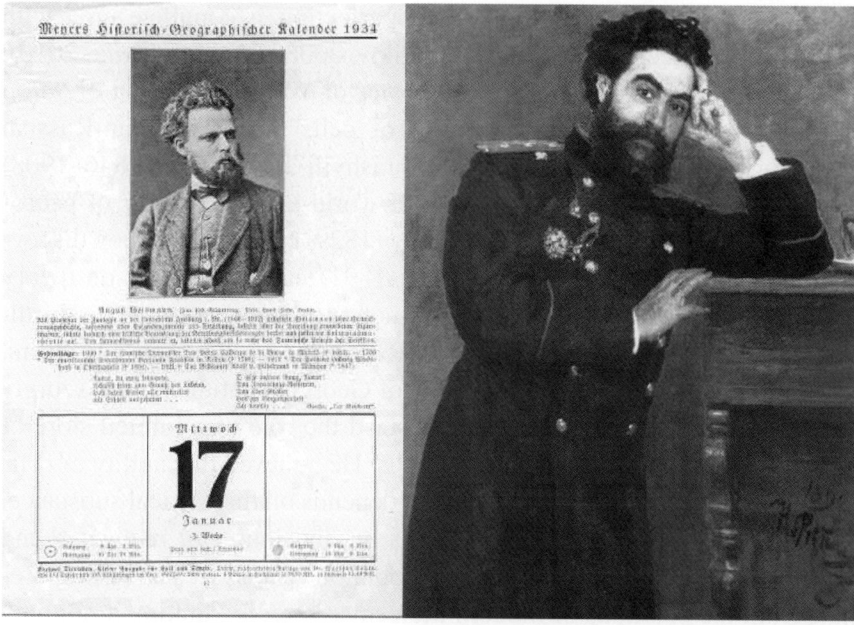

Figure 6.3. *Left*: Friedrich Leopold August Weismann (on calendar sheet, matching his centennial jubilee date) and his Russian follower in Gerontology prince Ivan R. Tarkhanov (Tarkhnishvili) — *Right* (portrait by I.E. Repin, oil/canvas, State Russian Museum, St. Petersburg).

limited). Weismann's concept, possibly, one of the most general and profound answers to a condemned question of medicine: "Why the reactivity of Homo did not give to it the absolutely perfect adaptations?" Such perfection is superfluous for the performance of reproductive duty, which Weismann considered to be the purpose of survival. Moreover, according to this point of view, it turns out that the chronic diseases, which in early phase do not interfere with accomplishing the task of reproduction, even may be evolutionarily advantageous to species, since they contribute to the change of generations. Therefore, natural selection to the interests of species had to support "delayed-action mine", i.e., those genetically determined features, which would be critical for the predisposition to such illnesses after the passing of the individual's reproductive age. The theory of disposable soma, serving just for needs of eternal germ cells had very profound impact on Russian biomedical science. We still interpret the whole pathophysiology as a science of body imperfection, in complete agree with Weismann's concept (Zaichik and Churilov, 2008; Churilov *et al.*,, 2010).

In Russian science of aging a follower of Weismann's idea of "drop in the limited reproductive potential of cells" was Georgian-Russian physiologist Ivan Ramazovich Tarkhnishvili-Tarkhanov (1846–1908) (Fig. 6.3, right). An eminent disciple of world-known founder of neurophysiology Ivan Mikhailovich Sechenov (1829–1905), Tarkhanov discovered the skin galvanic reflex, but later (1891) published work on theory of aging (Tarkhanov, 1891), which is not surprising, because his birthplace, Georgia, always was famous in Russia for numbers of long-livers. In his theory of aging direct descended of Georgian national hero Georgiy Saakadze, Prince Tarkhnishvili emphasized the role of a limited store of some "nuclear substance" within the cells. He believed that ability of cells to self-construction and to proliferation depends on this critical substance, which is shared between daughter cells on divisions, *not renovated* and step by step exhausted. In Tarkhanov's opinion (which we can now appreciate from the positions of modern molecular heredity, linking it not only to Weismann's view, but also to early ideas of British evolutionist Alfred Russell Wallace (1823–1913), aging it is not simple "wear of soma", but rather "decrement of nuclear substance" and loose of reparative, proliferating potencies in senile organism. At the same time, under the guidance of brilliant Russian clinician, Tarkhanov's friend: Sergei Petrovich Botkin (1832–1889), a group of Russian physicians performed first mass cohort study of elderly people in the history of medicine. In 1889 they made health screening of unique scale among 2620 old inhabitants of St, Petersburg hospices and described the results in a book (Kad'jan, 1890), published after Botkin's death by their team leader, medical doctor and revolutionary Alexander Alexandrovich Kad'jan (1849–1917). A lot of interesting correlations were revealed, perhaps, with world priority: like linkage between cataract and sclerosis of arteries, relation of non-diabetic microproteinuria to atherosclerosis and even connection between moderate drinking of vodka and better longevity. Hence, both S.P. Botkin and A.A. Kad'jan can be regarded as the founders of clinical gerontology in Russia and worldwide as well (Odin *et al.*, 2008) (Fig. 6.4).

A broadly generalized interdisciplinary approach to scientific problems, with an intermingle of the elements of natural science, philosophy and culture, was always characteristic for the Russian school of thinking.

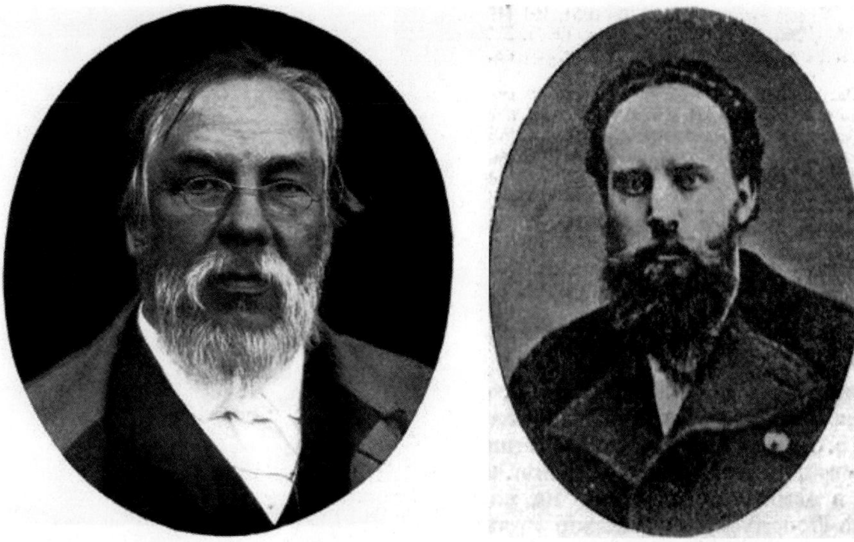

Figure 6.4. Teacher–Sergei Petrovich Botkin (*left*) and pupil — Alexander Alexandrovich Kad'jan — originators of Clinical Gerontology.

Whatever Russian mind goes in for — it always tends to create a world-view, that's why Russians are often great theorists, although much weaker inculcators. In full accordance with this statement, the roots of Russian Biogerontology of XX century can be found in teaching of Nikolai Feodorovich Feodorov (Gagarin) (1827–1903), an outstanding Orthodox Christian philosopher, early contributor to Russian *cosmism* doctrine and a precursor of transhumanism, which spread in Western thinking almost 70 years after Feodorov.

This thinker and futurologist (Fig. 6.5, left) was a bibliographer at Rumyantzev's museum library in Moscow. Teaching of Feodorov, this innate genius, was extremely important for all subsequent development of Russian civilization, including, of course, gerontology, and it needs to be detailed here. Feodorov opposed the very thought of authorship on books and ideas and, although his word sounded very authoritative among Russian intellectuals, during his lifetime he never published anything of written or said. Selection of his articles and letters was issued posthumously with the title "*Philosophy of the Common Task*" or "*Philosophy of Physical (Resuscitative) Resurrection*" (Feodorov, 1982).

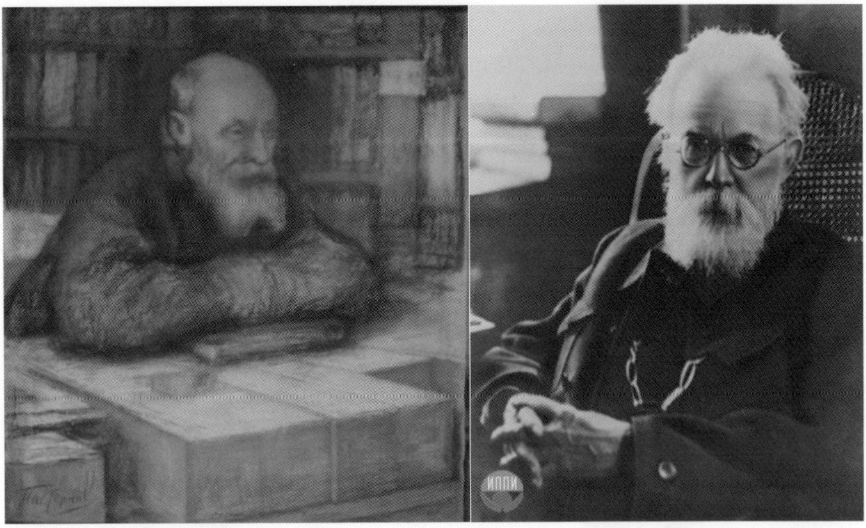

Figure 6.5. *Left*: Nikolai Feodorovich Feodorov (Gagarin), portrait by L.O. Pasternak and Vladimir Ivanovich Vernadskiy (*Right*).

According Feodorov, the human body is imperfect, but its evolution continues, which can lead to eventual perfection of the human race and society, including achievement of immortality with revival of the dead, and with Cosmos colonization. He argued that evolutionary process was directed towards increased intelligence and greater role of mind in the development of life. Homo is not only top product of evolution, but its moving force and director as well. Mankind must direct the next phases of evolution within the frames of its goals and under dictate of its morality. In Feodorov's opinion, *mortality* of humans is the most obvious indicator of the still *imperfect, contradictory* nature of Homo, the deep reason for most evil and nihilism of man and mankind. Feodorov combined in his doctrine the approach of natural science, which he considered to be the main caution to achieve immortality, and religious moral ideas of altruistic collectivism, deeply related to the Orthodox Christian understanding of Divine Trinity, united in three entities. There are two main reasons for mortality in Feodorov's opinion. One is endogenous imperfection of our body as regards to its material organization and functionality incapable of infinite self-renewal. To overcome this, scientifically-based psycho-physiological regulation of human organisms is needed. The second reason is exogenous: namely, the spontaneous nature of the external environment, its erratic character that must be overcome with global regulation "*introducing will and reason into nature*". This includes, according to Feodorov, prevention of natural disasters, control of Earth's climate, fight against epidemics, mastery of solar power, space exploration and ocean colonization. This is accomplishable only by a united mankind. But, according Feodorov's idea, it is the very struggle against death, which would become the most natural cause uniting all people of Earth, regardless of their nationality, cultural diversity, race, citizenship or wealth (he called this the "*Common Task*"). Feodorov interpreted resurrection not in purely religious way, but as a task for global science, its ultimate goal. He thought that death and post-mortem existence should become the subject of comprehensive scientific inquiry. And this knowledge must leave the laboratories and become the common property for all: "Everyone must be learning and everything be the subject of knowledge and action.... Our Body will become our Task" (in Russian "body" — "telo" and "Task" — "delo" sounds in rhyme, which makes last phrase sound like a slogan). According Feodorov's concept of "kinship", achieving immortality and resurrection of all people, who ever lived, are two inseparable goals, first is impossible to achieve, both ethically and physically, without achieving second one. We can't concede that our "kindred": ancestors, relatives and friends, who gave us life and culture, are missing dead. Kinship concept can be interpreted as early genetic idea. Feodorov taught that achieving immortality for living individuals and future generations is only a partial victory over death. The complete victory will come when everyone is returned to a *transformed* immortal life. He even planned specific actions for scientific research in this field. One of very fruitful thoughts of him was the idea of dissipation of body atoms after death and necessity to re-unite these elements of body *according program, existed in living individual* — for its resurrection. The subsequent development of trace elements doctrine and theory of biogenic migration of atoms by Russian naturalist and geochemist Vladimir Ivanovich Vernadskiy (1863–1945), father of Ecology, was directly inspired with Feodorov's philosophy (Fig. 6.5, right). Feodorov's first project was to collect and synthesize decayed remains of dead based on "knowledge and control over all atoms and molecules of the world". This idea of Feodorov stands very far ahead of his time and is related to the modern practice of cloning, which in fact represents organization of atoms according DNA program of a cloned organism. The next method prophesied by Feodorov was genetic-hereditary. The revival could be done successively in the ancestral line: sons and daughters restore their fathers and mothers; they in turn restore their parents and so on. This means restoring the ancestors using the hereditary information that they passed on to their children. But it is necessary also to give back into the revived person old mind and old epigenetic personality. Feodorov speculates about the existence of "radial images" that may contain the information about personalities of the people and continue to exist after their death. By mastering the forces of entropy and destruction, mankind will be able to "backup" the source of these images — physical individuals. Interestingly, the idea was to resurrect not a copy of existed imperfect body, but transform it into self-creating, mind-controlled form, immortal and capable of infinite renewal. Feodorov has sharpened the following paradox: in past people developed external technological tools, but their bodies stayed imperfect, which lead to discrepancy between the power of technology and weakness of the human organism. The transition is overdue from purely technical development, a "prosthetic" civilization, to organic progress, when organisms themselves are improved. This is the prototype of later idea of "biotechnology", which term was first coined much later, in 1930 by Russian zoologist and systemic biologist M.M. Zavadovskiy (1891–1957), who also was influenced much from Feodorov's doctrine. The philosopher made prognosis that Homo will be able to live in any environment, anticipating later V.I. Vernadsky's idea of an autotrophic man. Feodorov's genius originated many trends in Russian science, philosophy and arts.

We already mentioned ecology and its founder, a professor of St. Petersburg University, V.I. Vernadskiy. His doctrine of trace elements migration, as well as idea of ecological harmony and global ecological regulation for prerequisite of long healthy living can be regarded as contribution to gerontology. Moreover, the late book by Vernadskiy "*Thoughts of Naturalist: Space and Time in Alive and Non-alive Nature*" (Vernadskiy, 1975) contains very unusual ideas, for example, that the course of time within biological systems is subjective and can be physically accelerated (like in fever), or retarded (like in anabiosis). These ideas still wait for their experimental proof, but, in our opinion, they are wild enough to be the truth.

The world-recognized founder of cosmonautics, Konstantin Edwardovich Tsiolkovskiy (1857–1935), also was a direct disciple of Feodorov, attended his seminars and emphasized his influence ("*He has substituted University professors for me*"), especially as regards to ideas of cosmic expansion of Mankind. Hence, Feodorov's philosophy is a root of later Soviet breakthrough in space research.

In gerontology and geriatrics, direct inheritors of Feodorov's doctrine were Alexander A. Bogdanov (who also met Feodorov personally) and Alexander L. Chizhevskiy (direct disciple of Feodorov's pupil Tsiolkovsky). The brief description of their contribution to science of aging follows below. Even in last notes, written by outstanding Russian surgeon and anatomist, Nicolai Ivanovich Pirogov (1810–1881), whose bicentennial jubilee all Russia celebrated on November 25, 2010 (Fig. 6.6, left), as well as in last will expressed by great physician and executed by his pupils — one may

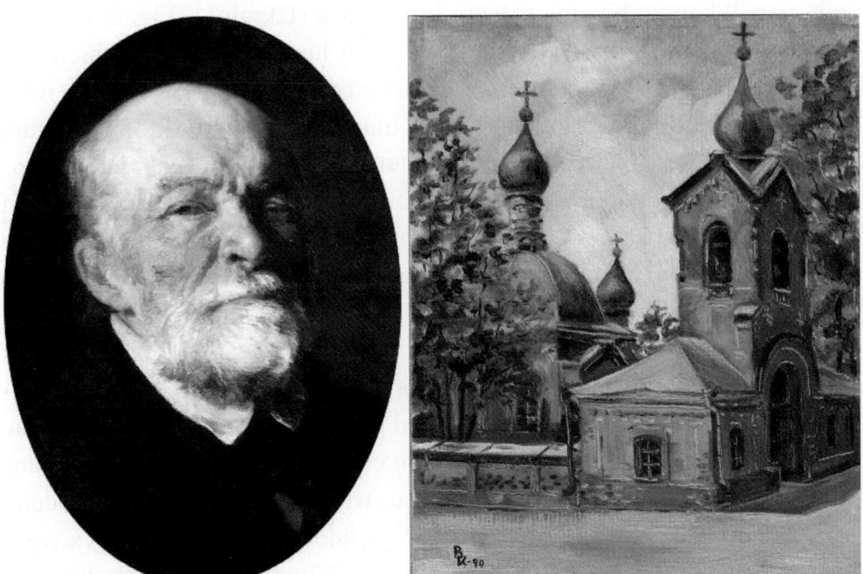

Figure 6.6. Nicolai Ivanovich Pirogov (Portrait by I.E. Repin, oil/canvas, State Russian museum, St. Petersburg) and Pirogov's mausoleum at his estate Vishnya in Vinnitsa, Ukraine (Picture by V.Ya. Kulakovskiy, oil/canvas, Yu.I. Stroev's private collection, St. Petersburg).

feel a deep kinship to Feodorov's concept. Pirogov, who was a scientist and physician, and quite rational in his way of thinking, stood far from hot religiosity. But he wrote in last days of his life on last pages of his famous "Notes of Old Physician" (Pirogov, 2008), "Yes, life — for me is a collective concept… Life — is the intelligent, limitlessly acting force, which controls all properties of substance …striving… to keep and support existence…. For the first time I wished immortality, post-mortem life. Love made this…. The faith into the immortality is based on something even higher than love itself. Now I believe in, or, it is more accurate to say, I desire the immortality not because of love only… no, my faith in the immortality is based now on other moral beginning, on other ideal." On these words Pirogov's diary was abrupt. Leading Russian medical scientist left this world with the thoughts of immortality. On December 5, 1881 at 20 h 25 min Pirogov died. Before his death he bequeathed to embalm and protect his body according the most up-to-date method by his disciple, Doctor D.I. Vyvodtsev, leading Russian specialist in that field. Pirogov's body is still kept at his mausoleum in Vinnitsa (Ukraine) (Fig. 6.5, right), and historians have discussed the reasons of his last decision, which was quite unusual for a Christian man. But we believe that he was influenced by Feodorov's doctrine and wanted to make easier the task of the future scientists, his possible resuscitators. Interestingly, many years later it was another pupil of Feodorov, eminent technical scientist, electric engineer, inventor and ambassador of USSR in Great Britain Leonid B. Krasin (1870–1926), who has convinced Soviet Government to embalm and protect the body of the founder of Soviet Union, V.I. Lenin (1870–1924). This project was realized by a team of leading anatomists and biochemists of that period. The great Russian philosopher of immortality and resurrection, Nicolai Feodorov, repeatedly said that only fundamental scientific studies of aging, death and post mortem conditions may reveal the means to overcome death. His skeptical phrase, well-known to Russian readers, is: "How unnatural would be to ask, 'Why does that, which exists, exist?' and yet how completely natural it is to ask, 'Why does the living die?"

If a reader will again look at the epigraph of this chapter above, it will be clear that another person, which also stood very close to Feodorov's philosophy, was Il'ya Il'ich Mechnikov, an associate professor of St. Petersburg University (Fig. 6.7). He was the founder of Russian experimental

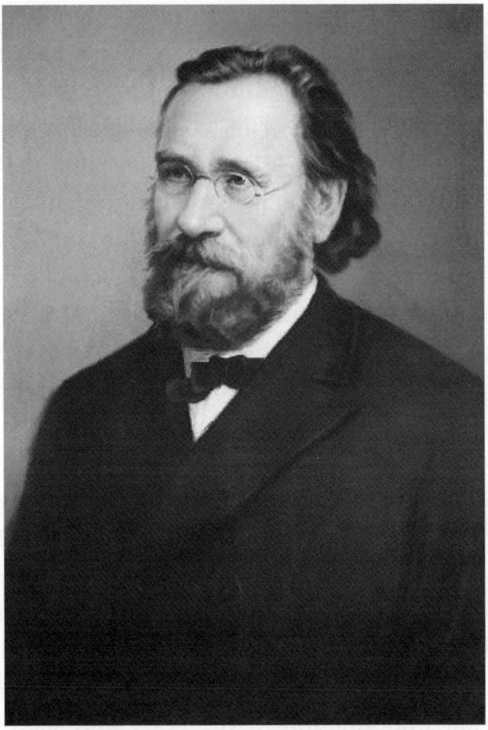

Figure 6.7. Il'ya Il'ich Mechnikov.

gerontology and *inventor of the very term Gerontology*, which he first coined in 1904 — see Metchnikoff (1903). Both Feodorov and Mechnikov considered mortality as a witness for disharmony of human nature, as well as they both interpreted the concept of human body imperfection. Initially Mechnikov's thoughts flowed within the trend of Weismann's "wear theory". Mechnikov had created the hypothesis, which treats the senile wear of organism as a result of autointoxication by the poisons of intestinal origin (Mechnikov, 1900). "*The reason for death — autointoxication of organism.... The longer are the bowels — the shorter is life*", he said in an aphoristic manner. Mechnikov regarded aromatic amines, formed by enteric bacteria, as the main toxicants; in order to decrease this vicious effect he has recommended constant consumption of sour-milk products containing living eubiotic microflora. His experiments showed the acceleration of senile changes in animals, getting indole and cresol derivates. Mechnikov introduced in world medicine the concept of "*orthobiosis*" — optimization of life conditions for its prolongation and healthy aging (distinct from premature). This concept keeps great popularity in practical geriatrics until now. Moreover, he insisted that many outdated adaptations and archetypical mechanisms, inherited by Homo from its evolutionary ancestors, are no longer optimal for conditions of human living and serve as a source of our imperfection. Mechnikov changed the paradigm in the field of longevity studies — from the narrow field of hygienic recommendations to the broad basis of general and evolutionary biology. To understand entirely all fruitful potential of his aging theory, we need to remember that he also was a founder of the concept of "*physiological (regulatory) autoimmunity*." As early as in 1892 I.I. Metchnikoff published a small paper on the existence of Darwinian struggle between cellular elements of the same Metazoan organism (Metchnikoff, 1892). According his idea, immunity and the specialized cells responsible for it are evolutionary necessary, first of all not as warriors against aliens but in order to keep peace within self-body by means of harmonization of the contradictions between its elements. In this fruitful concept immune system looks like product of inherent imperfection of the body and serves for permanent self–construction and remodeling of the self-organism in ontogenesis, by means of "*physiological inflammation*" or (as it was named by Mechnikov and his pupils later) — "*natural autoimmunity*". Unfortunately, his lone voice was not heard at that time, and it was only much later that similar ideas were expressed. For a long time, practically, from the moment of its origination (1900), the classical immunology, regarding the problem of autoimmunity, was adhered to a principle of «*Horror autotoxicus*», attributed to P. Ehrlich and E. Morgenroth (Poletaev and Churilov, 2010). This concept claims that no antibodies can be formed against self-components in healthy organism. Almost immediately after its declaration, I.I. Mechnikov's disciple (later a professor of St. Petersburg University), Yefim Semyonovich London (1901) has obtained in experiment the auto-antibodies against human sperm and demonstrated their presence in sera of *healthy* men (London, 1901). Another Mechnikov's pupil Alexander M. Besredka has registered the existence of *natural* autoantibodies towards self red blood cells (1901) (Poletaev and Churilov, 2010).

Although the dogma of purely pathological essence of autoimmunity has been shaken, but not broken, still the immunologists believed that autoimmune response is illegal and possible only in experiments and in disease. This statement with minor changes was still in use until late 1970s. It is conceptually important that such an unilateral attitude to autoimmunity, reproduced even by some recently published textbooks and attributed to Paul Ehrlich's name, in fact has not any basis in P. Ehrlich's papers. On the contrary, P. Ehrlich has anticipated the modern concept of physiological autoimmunity, because he regarded antibodies as a kind of circulating cellular receptors, disattached from a cell surface (Metchnikoff and Rue, 1914), thus expecting the homology between receptor proteins and autoantibodies.

Basically, as double-stranded DNA encodes the genetic programs of an organism, it is obvious that opposite to any peptide its structural antonym or anti-peptide should be encoded. It means that the ability to generate anti-signals and anti-receptors is deep-seated into the intrinsic fundament of cell regulation (Smith *et al.*, 1987). From this standpoint the phrase "Body consists of Anti-Bodies" looks not like figurative, but almost literal one. Much earlier this was brightly expressed in ancient Chinese pictogram of Yin/Yang confluence.

Mechnikov and his school also interpreted cellular autoimmunity as a physiological one. The phenomenon of phagocytosis was discovered by Mechnikov in 1883, and since then many representatives of biomedicine treated this process (borrowed as function of endocellular digestion from Protozoa) as the protective reaction peculiar to the pathological conditions and directed only against the non-self, alien objects. Nevertheless, the founders of immunology themselves have established that cellular mechanisms of autoaggression are inherent to a healthy organism. Mechnikov and his co-worker AO. Kovalevskiy emphasized, that during early ontogeny cells of provisional organs in fly larvae are eliminated by own wandering phagocytes (Metchnikoff, 1902).

Quite early on, Mechnikov has assumed that autoantibodies provide a senile atrophy of the organs, and self macrophages of stromal, mesenchymal origin may attack "noble", highly specialized elements of organs' parenchyma in self tissues, thus promoting not only physiological cell renewal, but (in their excessive activity) — also senile fibrosis, sclerosis or gliosis, registered as aging (Metchnikoff, 1901). However the phenomenon of autophagocytosis, making a basis for morphogenesis and differentiation, remained without proper attention for many decades, almost until 1981–1984, when M.M.B. Kay demonstrated that physiological programmed cell elimination in ontogeny may be caused by natural autoimmune response to non-tissue-specific glycoprotein band-III (antigen of senescent cells), expressed on their surface (Kay, 1983). Natural physiological autoantibodies mark the cells which have to be eliminated, and self-macrophages carry out their opsonin-dependent phagocytosis — in full accordance with Mechnikov's prediction, made 80 years before these experiments. Nowadays many researchers pay attention to autophagocytosis and autoagressive behavior of glial cells in such an important geriatric illness as Alzheimer's disease. Hence, Mechnikov was the first scientist who linked senescence to autoimmunity exaggerated to the degree of autoallergy, and interpreted it as a result of conflict between self tissues (changed due to autointoxication), and self-reactive mesenchymal cells (excessively stimulated by toxins), attacking the "noble" elements with autophagocytosis and autoantibodies. This idea was deeply implanted in his disciples and produced long lasting consequences for the Russian school of gerontology. Among the scientists of Mechnikov's school, both interest in gerontological problems and activity in the field of autoimmunity have always co-existed. Mechnikov had graduated from University of Khar'kov (1865). Much later the same school conferred M.D. Diploma upon another graduate, whose destiny was to promote greatly gerontology, blood transfusion and cybernetics in Russia and to facilitate the development of both Feodorov's and Mechnikov's ideas. It was prominent Russian polymath Alexander Alexandrovich Bogdanov (aka: Malinovskiy, 1873–1928) (Fig. 6.8). Bogdanov was a very versatile and talented person. Being a medical doctor with specialization in psychiatry, he wrote (1913–1923) one of the first books in protocybernetics with the original formulation of general systems theory, foremost in the world science: "*Essays in Tektology. The General Science of Organization*" (Bogdanov, 1980). He is also recognized as one of the founders of scientific management, eminent sociologist, relativistic philosopher, science fiction writer and futurologist, and has forecasted many phenomena of modern life (beginning from computers and atomic bomb — and ending with sexual revolution, euthanasia

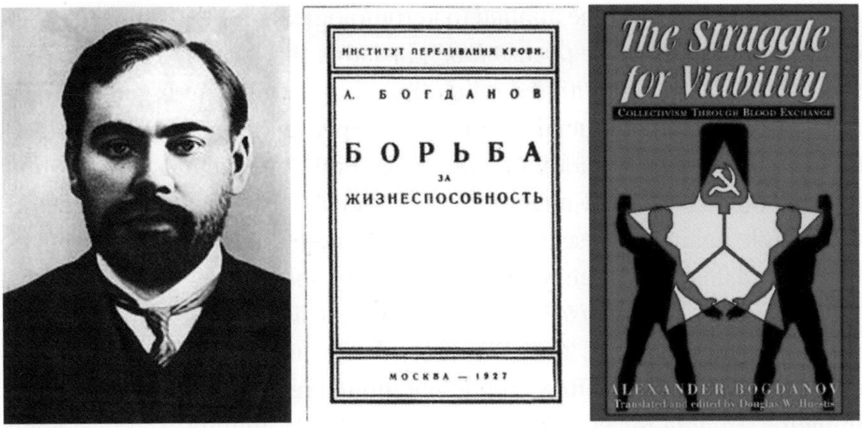

Figure 6.8. Alexander Alexandrovich Bogdanov; covers of 1st (1927) and latest American (2002) editions of his main medical book "The Struggle for Viability".

clinics and global role of English language). He was an active and influential Bolshevist revolutionary, a close friend of Lenin, and suggested the Red Star as the Soviet symbol, although after the victory of Bolshevism in Russia, Bogdanov stopped any political activity due to his very critical attitude to Lenin's model of communism (Tjukin *et al.*, 2010). For medical science, including gerontology, it was very happy occasion, because such a unique mind concentrated entirely on experimental and organizational medical work and achieved many results in very short period (1917–1928), being supported by Soviet leaders, who trusted to his medical ideas, in spite of distrust to his philosophy. Bogdanov, in fact, was first Soviet gerontologist: he created original cybernetic theory of aging and founded first Soviet laboratory, systematically working in the field of experimental gerontology. According his Tektology doctrine, or version of General Systems Theory, the reason of senescence is diminishing of body's integrity, or growing contradiction between the interests of a whole organism and its differentiating parts, with a kind of dissynchronization in ontogeny of different organs. He formulated the principle of so-called *egression*. According this principle, complex hierarchical systems with time shift to prevail of central regulatory influences, which makes them less plastic and decrease their resistance. So, he interpreted senescence as general phenomenon, an exemplary case to egression. Also he applied to gerontological problems the tektological principle of a "*loose (weak) link*", insisting that general reliability of a senile body is limited with the reliability of a less resistant organ or tissue. A candidate for this crucial role in senescence in his opinion was blood, as a tissue carrying humoral (endocrine and immune) signals, establishing the communication and integrity of body elements. Bogdanov suggested to struggle against senescence by means of hemotransfusions or even via blood exchange between young and elderly individuals. He called that "*physiological collectivism*" and proposed that such a treatment will allow the individuals to share their reactivity, for example, through antibodies contained in blood, and may strengthen mutual resistance of the organisms in their "*struggle for viability*" (Bogdanov, 2002). Initially, the idea about the curativeness of blood transfusions came to Bogdanov, when he studied protozoology at the Khar'kov University, which was being famous for its school of protistologists, founded by the discoverer of lambliasis Dushan F. Lamble (1824–1895). Bogdanov's attention drew the phenomenon of the conjugation, when unicellular organisms "rejuvenate", being exchanged with the parts of cytoplasm (as we now know, with DNA of plasmids). By analogy with this, Bogdanov assumed that the exchange of the blood can render the effect of rejuvenating and strengthening body resistance. Later, in studentship he experienced strong influence from Feodorov and Tsiolkovskiy (both of them he has met personally) and was impressed with rapid development of serology, serotherapy and immunology, including the ideas of isohemagglutination discoverer I.I. Mechnikov and the first achievements of K. Landsteiner's blood group theory. As an energetic and talented practical organizer, Bogdanov created the Moscow Institute of Blood Transfusion, the first worldwide, with an Experimental Unit headed by closest pupil of Mechnikov, Alexander Alexandrovich Bogomolets (1881–1946) (Fig. 6.9). Besides the unique role of this Institution in blood banking and development of national blood transfusion service (because to it USSR became world leading country in this field and entered into WW II with excellent Transfusiology) (Huestis, 2007), it is worth mentioning that the Experimental unit and A.A. Bogomolets personally worked on the basis of Bogdanov's gerontological ideas (Bogdanoff, 1927). Regrettably, the originator of this trend in Soviet gerontology, A.A. Bogdanov, perished in 1928 as a result of a risky experiment performed on himself. He was

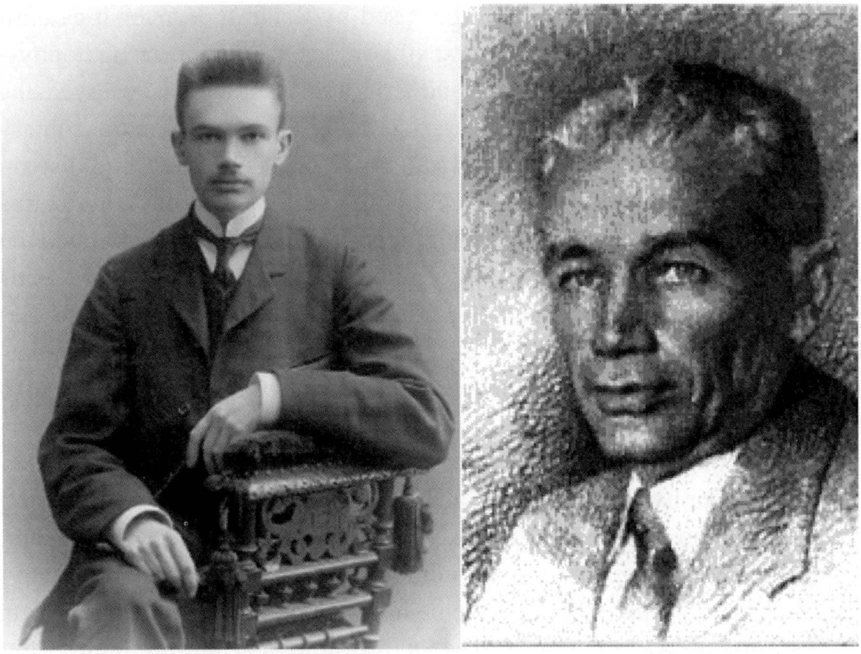

Figure 6.9. Alexander Alexandrovich Bogomoletz, *left* — Mechnikov's student, *right* — Soviet academician.

making group-compatible exchanging blood transfusion with a young tuberculosis patient, Lev Koldomasov, in an attempt to save him. Unfortunately, the Rh-system was discovered much later — in 1940 (Tjukin *et al.*, 2010). Rhesus-positive Koldomasov recovered, but rhesus-negative Bogdanov died from acute renal failure, caused by Rh-conflict (which manifestations he described in his last self-observation). He left a son, Alexander Alexandrovich Malinovskiy (junior) (1909–1996), who was a weak and subtle kid, but recovered after hemotransfusion treatment, growing up to become an eminent systemic biologist and genetist, and an active and long-living gerontologist. The son developed in aging science the systemic approach and cybernetic ideas of his father (Malinovskiy, 1986).

After Bogdanov's death a relay of frontiers in Soviet Gerontology was taken by A.A. Bogomolets (Fig. 6.9) and his school. Bogomolets was by far the most noticeable Soviet pathophysiologist, who created the very system of pathophysiology teaching, used by domestic universities until now, and wrote the first domestic textbook and workshop in pathophysiology. He was an experimental endocrinologist, and first observed the universal response of the adrenocortical cells to different extraordinary stimuli. Also he predicted the lipid nature of their hormones, and discovered the stimulating action of anticellular ("cytotoxic") immunoglobulins on the endocrine cells (1909) (Bogomolets, 1909). Later he formulated the original concept and classification of human somatotypes, based on various properties of active mesenchyma and preponderance of certain types of connective tissue in bodies of different individuals (1926). Bogomolets transformed gerontological concept of his teacher, Mechnikov. He also was adept of physiological autoimmunity concept. Moreover, many experimental proofs of cell function and growth stimulation by means of tissue-specific antisera or autoantibodies were obtained by him and later on by his numerous disciples (Zaichik *et al.*, 2008). But, unlike his teacher, he did not emphasize the role of conflict between "inferior" mesenchymal and "noble" parenchymal elements in gerontogenesis. Bogomolets instead insisted on regulating role of physiological autoimmunity and put the connective tissue in the center of healthy gomeodynamics of the organism, definitely under the influence of Bogdanov's "weak link" principle. He stated that, "A person has the age of his/her connective tissue" (Bogomolets, 1940). Several other precursors of Bogomolets' theory of aging, quoted by him, were Swiss organic chemist Amé Pictet (1867–1937), who assumed (Pictet, 1916) that the basis of body wear is the progressive cyclization of aliphatic chemical bounds in the organism, which impedes their solubility and metabolism; and also Rumanian neuropathologist George Marinesco (1863–1938) (Marinesco, 1928) (who by the way severely criticized Mechnikov's idea of "autophagocytic attack" against the nobles of body). Marinesco instead, since 1919, had studied the protein colloids of the brain, turning attention to their dehydration and reduction in degree of their dispersiveness, which he considered as the main aging mechanism. The inventor of cinematography Auguste Lumièr (1862–1954), man of wide scientific interests, while checking the wear of movie picture films, expressed one brilliant guess (Lumière, 1921), that the wear of living tissues during senescence can be explained by the analogous "flocculation of the long-life biocolloids" of the body. And finally, Czech pathophysiologist and geneticist Vladimir T. Ružicka (1922) modified all these concepts and introduced an idea about "*protoplasmic hysteresis*", i.e., gradual packing, dehydration, coagulation and a decrease of cytoplasmic protein solubility in the course of aging. Bogomolez implanted the results of synthesis of these concepts into the soil of Mechnikov's and Bogdanov's imaginations; and developed the theory of "*age-related colloidoclazia*" (1940). Under this name he understood the flocculation of cellular and intercellular matrix colloids, first of all — the denaturizing of the connective tissue proteins, without their adequate proteolysis (Bogomoles, 1940). This, on his thought, must alter the homeostasis, which requires the intercellular exchange with substrata and signals. For experimental therapy of aging, aimed to colloidoclasia, Bogomolets proposed polyclonal antibodies against the connective tissue — antireticular cytotoxic serum (ACS). This serum has stimulated the immunity, reparation and functions of macrophages and was broadly used in the USSR (1937–1980) as immunostimulator, wound healing remedy and life prolongation agent. For many years after his passing, the city of Kyiv, where he worked for a long period, became the center of Soviet aging science, with its academic Research Institute of Gerontology and Geriatrics established there in 1940. Bogomolets originated in Russian science very strong tradition of searching the links between autoimmunity and biogerontological problems. His closest disciple, Leonid R. Perelman (1900–1969) coined in an idea of using specific antisera against different subcellular fractions in order to separate cytotoxic and cytostimulating effects of ACS and similar antibodies (Perelman, 1966). The closest pupil of Perelman, Albert Sh. Zaichik and his co-workers, practically achieved that and experimentally confirmed that antibodies towards some chromatin antigens of endocrine cells are devoid of cytolytic effect, but possess with very strong ability to stimulate hormone production and some mitogenic potential for target cells (Poletaev and Churilov, 2010; Zaichik *et al.*, 2008). It has been shown that different specific antibodies penetrate *in vivo* into target cell nuclei, stimulate RNA biosynthesis and target cell hormone production — which is the true for anti-thyroid, anti-adrenocortical and anti-pituitary antinuclear IgG. Autoantibodies of similar specificity were repeatedly registered in sera of intact animals and healthy individuals. Cytostimulating antibodies (but not pre-immune ones) were even able to substitute pituitary tropic hormones for adrenal cortex and induce hypertrophy of target organ on chronic repeated injections. Moreover, apoptosis by default, starting in target peripheral endocrine glands after pituitary removal, could be retarded by means of specific anti-nuclear immunoglobulins. Interestingly, the inhibition of adrenal glands atrophy was also observed in hypophysectomized animals under the influence of actinomycin D. It testified for this kind of atrophy in itself represents the programmed process demanding the reference to genetic matrixes and needed in some RNAs biosynthesis. Delay of this programmed atrophy could be observed not only under the influence of specific IgG, but also under the condition of hypothyroidism (Zaichik *et al.*, 2008). These studies facilitated a bridge making between autoimmune and endocrine aspects of senescence (see below). In its current interpretation, the autoimmune concept of senescence underlines two aspects.

At first, the systems supervising growth, development and aging of the whole organism and all its components have to coordinate sequence and intensity of reading and realization of the genetic information in various cells. This task can not be achieved neither by neural mechanisms, nor via hormonal agents, which are accelerating or slowing down the metabolic processes. The neurotransmitters, hormones and their receptors will not suffice ontogenetic and event-driven variability for this purpose; the cells which produce them are devoid of necessary mobility and all-embracing dispersal. But these are qualities inherent to immune system. Genetically determined events defining a maturity of regulatory and metabolic systems at every stage of ontogeny should occur in coordinated manner within various organs and tissues. They cannot be carried out in the contrary with the universal "law of reflection". The system of physiological autoimmunity serves as a mirror in dynamic maintenance of individual self-identity, because it is capable of universal inducible reproduction of complementary molecules. The network of idiotype-antiidiotypic regulation includes receptors of hormones, autacoids and neurotransmitters, as well as auto-antiidiotypic antibodies to all these bioregulators, which in turn, are mirror «internal immunological images» of their ligands (Zaichik *et al.*, 2008; Poletaev and Churilov, 2010). In our opinion, the bioregulators developed by immune system carry out the function of "pointing fingers" in process of coordinated gene expression for various cells of an organism. Auto-reactive molecules can play a repressor, or vice versa — derepression role for certain sites of genome, not allowing dyscoordinated differentiation and desynchronization in senescence of various organs and tissues. Evidently, the interaction of immunoglobulins with information systems of stem cells defines an orientation of their differentiation processes throughout the whole life cycle, since the prenatal period of ontogeny. There are numerous experimental works, mostly by Russian authors, on the mitogenic effects of autoantibodies and on the phenomenon of organospecific stimulation of regeneration by means of passive transfer of immunoglobulins from a donor animal, which had an injury of an organ in reparative phase, to a recipient animal without organ injury (Zaichik and Churilov, 2008). The comprehensive review of these data from gerontological point of view was given by Dontsov (1998), a substantial contributor to this field. Thus, physiological autoimmunity normally may provide bringing-together and co-tuning of genetic information reading in different cells of the holistic "Body" through the whole life, and during physiological senescence — as well.

At second, we shall not forget that process of senescence can be accelerated up to premature aging rates. And in this phenomenon the role of autoimmunity exaggerated to autoallergy is also significant. Below we will discuss some data on immunoendocrine disorders causing accelerated aging, and our own studies on this matter.

The tree of domestic gerontology, although it is very young, is comparable to the long-living trees from Jingshan Gongyuan park in Beijing or sequoias of Washington state (Fig. 6.10), and has many branches besides the main trunks described above. Among the most important achievements of Russian gerontology we shall mention few more interesting experimental results and theoretical considerations.

One branch is related to biophysical approach of rejuvenation. A pupil of Tsiolkovskiy, eminent biophysicist and pathophysiologist Alexander Leonidovich Chizhevskiy (1897–1964), founder of Heliobiology, discovered influence of solar activity on biological and biosocial processes on the Earth (1924). Later, in search for the mechanisms mediating these effects, he explored the influence of atmospheric aeroions on vital activity and lifespan of experimental animals (1936). It appeared that negatively charged aeroions improved health and prolonged life of animals. In contrast, complete isolation from geomagnetic field shortened their life

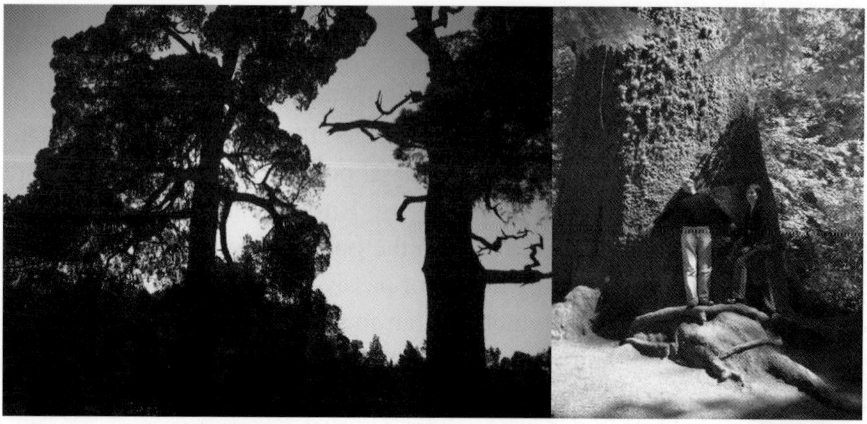

Figure 6.10. *Left*: 1100 years old cypress trees at Jingshan Gongyuan. *Right*: 550 years old "Monarch" sequoia in USA (Photos by authors). In the world of plants the enigma of longevity is already solved.

(Chizhevsky, 1976). The contemporaries called this polymath scholar, successor of Russian cosmism, "Soviet Leonardo" (Fig. 6.11). Chizhevskiy inculcated his discoveries into communal hygiene and the practice of physiotherapy though the "Aeroionification Program of the USSR", which obtained broad state support. Scientific supervisor of the construction of the Palace of Soviets at Moscow, nominee for Nobel Prize, President Emeritus of the 1st World Congress of 1939 in Biophysics and Cosmic Biology at New York, and later, a scientist falsely accused in anti-Soviet conspiracy and imprisoned (1942). An air ionizing device, invented by him (Chizhevskiy's chandelier), is still very popular among Russian physiotherapists and patients.

Equally strong was the Soviet biochemical branch of gerontology. Today one of the topics of intensive research worldwide is a role of SIR-genes (sirtuins) in longevity (Sinclair and Guarente, 2006). It has been proven that sirtuins' expression is induced by several factors, including a lean diet. In this regards we have a pleasure to mention that pioneering work, which for the first time registered the life-prolonging effect of a lean diet in an animal model, was made as early as in 1914 in Russia by a zoologist from St. Petersburg (later — Khar'kov) Universities. E.A. Schultz demonstrated in Hydrae and Planariae that periodical starvation improves

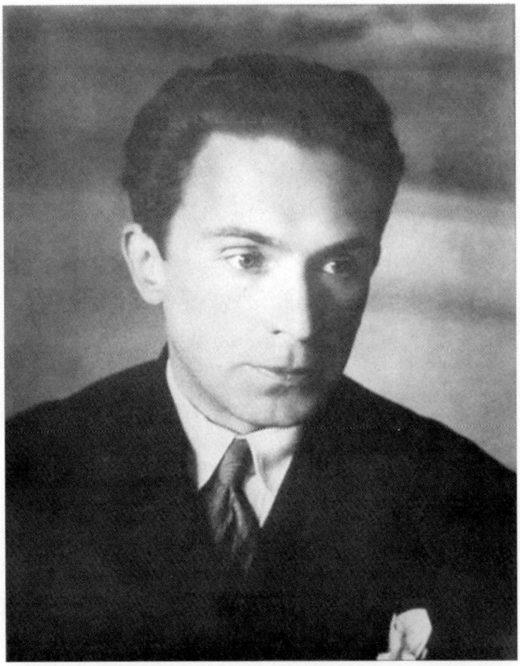

Figure 6.11. Alexander Leonidovich Chizhevskiy, "Soviet Leonardo."

the regeneration processes and elongates lifespan of these Invertebrate (Schultz, 1914). In Western countries this concept's origin is calculated from the later publication of Osborn (Osborn *et al.*, 1917). The senescence in the opinion of many theoreticians and experimental scientists was tightly related to the "tempo of living", sometimes interpreted as amount of genetically determined events per unite of time, sometimes — as a speed of metabolism. German physiologist Max Rubner (1854–1932) coined in an idea in 1908 that longevity depends on total energy expenditure and, thus on basic metabolic rate and oxygen consumption (we shall note, that role of thyroid gland in control of these parameters was already under his suspicions) (Rubner, 1908). Russian geriatrist and physiotherapist Abram (aka: Alexander) Solomonovich Zalmanov (1875–1965) (Fig. 6.12) interpreted the linkage between senescence and oxygen as a necessity of balance in oxygen supply and supply of substrates of oxidation (Zalmanov, 1966). This is in accordance with much later studies on complete and

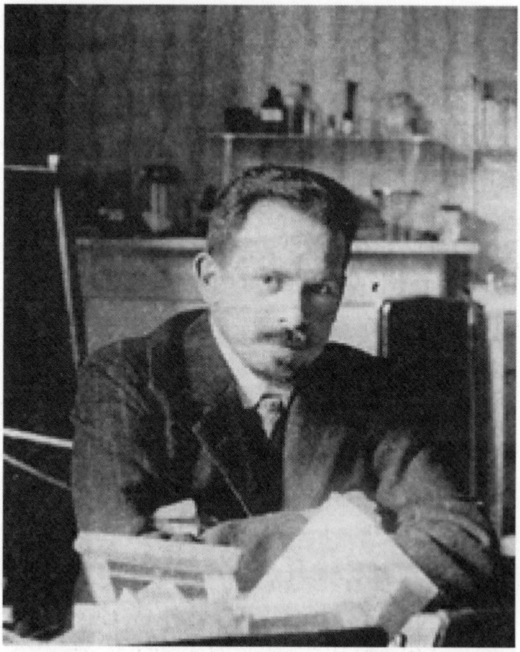

Figure 6.12. Abram Solomonovich Zalmanov.

non-complete reduction of oxygen and relation of non-complete reduction to production of free radicals, proven agents of senescence (Harman, 1956). As a caution to establish such a balance, Zalmanov, being a practitioner and influenced from last fashion in physiology of that time — microcirculation studies of Danish scientist August Krogh — has recommended activation of microcirculation ("capillary wash") by means of well-known inducer of arterial hyperemia — turpentine oil. The Zalmanov's turpentine baths became popular method of vital tonus support and even pretended to facilitate rejuvenation, at least for skin. It is worth to mention, that activation of microcirculation in thyroid, achieved by Zalmanov's method, could improve its function in geriatric patients. A.S. Zalmanov was the private Kremlin doctor of Soviet leader V.I. Lenin. Even after emigration to France, later occupied by Nazi, Zalmanov kept Soviet citizenship. World fame came to him, when in 1958 he has broadly published a geriatric book with description of his concept and method: "*Secrets and Wisdom of Human Body*". The interpretation of senescence and degeneration of living tissues as a result of broadly understood "undernourishment" or "chronic partial starvation" (including not only substrate, but also oxygen deficiency) was deeply rooted in domestic gerontology, beginning from Zalmanov's concept and later "bioreduction theory" developed by eminent pathomorphologist from Baku, disciple of Rudolf Virchow, Moisey Solomonovich Müehlman (1867–1940). Müehlman authored one of the first Soviet monographs in theoretical biogerontology (1926, later translated in German) (Müehlman, 1927), where he interpreted senescence as a result of growth and related insufficiency of tissue nutrition and vital components supply. Even long after Müehlman's book Russian gerontologists always took into account the fundamental role of hypoxia as most frequent typical pathologic process accompanying every case of death, every event of cell necrobiosis, at least in the final phase, and quite often existing from the very beginning of a lethal disease. Thus, since hypoxia is the most wide-spread pathological process always accompanying acute death, the stress, which improves the resistance to acute hypoxia, will adapt the organism nonspecifically to a large number of various influences. That is why the term "nonspecific resistance" is *de facto* understood as an "anti-hypoxic resistance" (Zaichik and Churilov, 2008). Due to such considerations, thoughts on possible links between hypoxia, antihypoxic resistance, adaptation to hypoxia, senescence and rejuvenation, were born in the minds of several eminent domestic pathophysiologists.

First of all we need to mention among them Nikolai Nikolaevich Sirotinin (1896–1977). According his conception, ontogenesis is the process of asynchronous expression and repression of the unfolding genetic programs. That is why individuals of different ages have different reactivity. Sirotinin established on the mountain of Elbrus, the highest in Europe, an experimental laboratory involved in pathophysiology of hypoxia and ontogenesis of human reactivity (Fig. 6.13). He made also comparative zoological studies as regards to evolution of anti-hypoxic adaptation. His works were of great applied value in aerospace medicine; he made outstanding contribution in research of high altitude disease, invented stepwise principle of mountain acclimatization and gaseous mixtures for prevention of hypoxia and hypocapnia under extreme conditions. Due to all that he was the single pathophysiologist, ever awarded "K.E. Tsiolkovskiy's Medal",

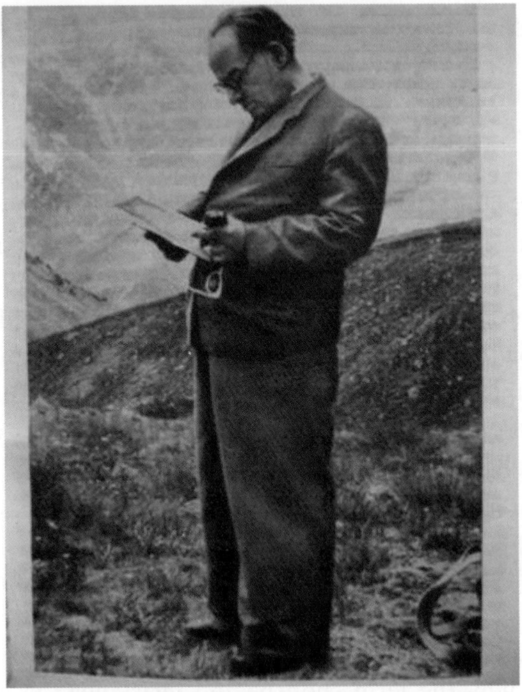

Figure 6.13. Nicolai Nicolaevich Sirotinin during experiments on himself on the mountain of Elbrus.

handed only to cosmonauts and astronauts. Sirotinin experimentally proved that anti-hypoxic resistance of the organism in acute hypoxia is inversely depending on age (Sirotinin, 1981). This is known as "*Sirotinin's rule*": immature cells and earlier ontogenetic stages of any vertebrate of invertebrate organism are more resistant to acute hypoxia, than mature or later ones (for example, fetus and neonate in humans survive in acute hypoxia for longer time than adults, and elderly adults have even less survival rate). There are now many mechanisms discovered which are responsible for this phenomenon. These are specific phosphofructokinases of immature cells, less prone to acidic inhibition, fetal hemoglobin, more affine to oxygen, different patterns of hypoxic stress reaction in adult and immature adrenals etc. (Zaichik and Churilov, 2008). And nowadays every flight attendant, when instructing air passengers to put oxygen mask on adults first, and on kids last, exploits the discovery of this Russian scientist. Gerontological extraction, made by him from these experiments was the idea of stepwise hypoxic training in order to stimulate some shift of metabolism within the elderly and mature tissues — to juvenile patterns, evolutionary more appropriate for hypoxic conditions. Sirotinin has shown that combination of moderate hypoxia with hypercapnia and hypothermia decreases the pathogenic potential of hypoxic factor and elicits in cells some archetypical ancient mechanisms of adaptation, which may increase the resistance of body to many different pathogenic agents, besides the hypoxia itself. He related this to the phylogeny of the ancient mechanisms of hibernation in animals and to problem of anabiosis as a method of life conservation and prolongation (Sirotinin, 1981). Moreover, if one will reverse Sirotinin's rule, it will appear that resistance to hyperoxia (or, the same — to oxidative stress) in immature organism is lower, than in mature one. This may be concretized for resistance to any free-radical producing pathogenic factor, for example — to chlorine-organic toxicants or even to ionizing radiation, because main mechanism of its action is free-radical stress via radiolysis of intracellular water (Zaichik and Churilov, 2008). Long before Sirotinin (in 1905) French radiobiologists have noticed that radiosensitivity of cells and tissues is inversely dependant on the degree of their maturity and directly proportional to their mitotic rates, which is known as "*Rule of Bergonier–Tribondeau*" (Bergonier and Tribondeau, 1905). In fact, now we can interpret both rules as two sides of the same coin: ontogeny or aging means progressive loss of anti-hypoxic potential, and from the very beginning, the body has high, although diminishing, sensitivity to hyperoxia and free oxidative radicals (Zaichik and Churilov, 2008)! To finalize the discussion of ideas, grown up around the relation of oxygen and senescence in Russian gerontology, we need to mention that, although world priority of Denham Harman's work on senescence as auto-oxidation goes without saying (Harman, 1956), the scientist, who received the 1956 Nobel prize for the discovery and theory of free-radical chain reactions, was a professor of Leningrad (now St. Petersburg) University Nicolai Nicolaevich Semyonov (1896–1986), whose publications (Semyonov, 1935), of course, were known to chemical technologist Harman, were quoted by him and influenced on his search (Harman, 1956). Two years after Harman's analogous theory of senescence was developed for polymers and biological

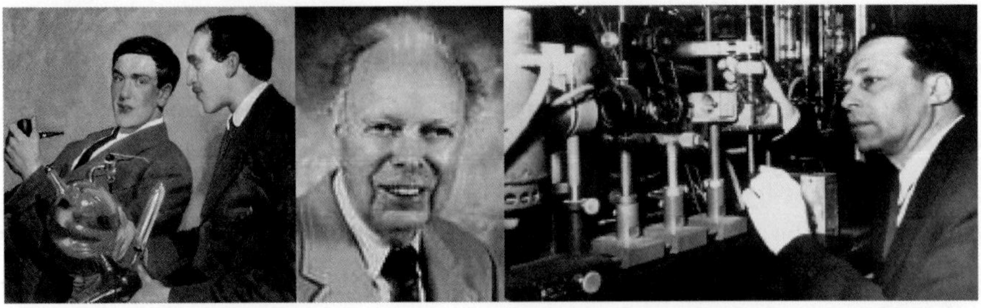

Figure 6.14. *Left photo*: Nicolai Nicolaevich Semyonov in student years (Right, left one is another future Soviet Noble Prize winner — Pyotr Leonidovich Kapitsa). Portrait by B.M. Kustodiev, oil/canvas. Kapitsa collection, Moscow. Most outstanding thing is that to the moment when this portrait was made (1921), both young postgraduates were absolutely not known, not able to pay to the artist of Kustodiev's level properly — and he rejected their custom, saying: "I paint either very rich, or very famous people!", and finally, after their promise to achieve fame in future, agreed to do this job as a matter of exclusion and took in compensation from 2 youngsters… a rooster. Many years later both Nicolai and Pyotr executed the promise given to painter and became world famous Noble Prize laureates. On the *middle photo* — Denham A. Harman (Born 1916), alive classic of oxidative stress doctrine of senescence, applied follower of Semyonov's fundamental research. *Right photo* — Nikolai Markovich Emanuel, Soviet researcher of free radical mechanisms of aging.

gels by Semyonov's disciple, Soviet physico-chemist Nikolai Markovich Emanuel (1915–1984) (Emanuel, 1985). All these contributors of free radical theory can be seen in Fig. 6.14. Contemporary Russian biochemist V.P. Skulachev is a direct descendant of this school, because his research correlated senescence and apoptosis to mitochondrion function, free radical production and oxygen consumption in cells. He coined in the word "phenoptosis", as a term for programmed involution of the whole body (Skulachev, 2003). He hypothesized that by means of decrease of free radical levels in mitochondria it would be possible to retard the realization of phenoptotic program and transition of free radical apoptogenic signals from cell to cell. Skulachev *et al.* suggested antioxidants of a new type called SkQ — cationic quinones, able to intramitochondrial penetration. Experiments have shown their effectiveness in some senile diseases. Moreover, species with intensive aerobic metabolism may have natural methionine–related protective analogues of such mechanism in their mitochondria (Skulachev *et al.*, 2009).

Fundamental chemistry, physics and chemical physics were highly developed in Russia to the beginning of 20th century, due to efforts of periodic law originator D. I. Mendeleev (1834–1907), inventor of radio A.S. Popov (1859–1906), discoverer of photonic pressure P.N. Lebedev (1866–1912), and other world-known scientists. That's why Russian and later Soviet Biomedicine from the first steps had very substantial physical and chemical basis and obvious bias to fundamental natural sciences. For example, it was Russian pathophysiologist Ye.S. London (1869–1938), mentioned above, who has pioneered the biomedical studies of radium and its effects on the organism, including rates of aging, produced the first experimental model of radiation sickness and invented the method of autoradiography, now broadly used worldwide. This scientist also published first in world science monograph in radiobiology (London, 1911) and by personal letter convinced Tsar Nicholas II to purchase abroad huge amount of radium in order to supply and promote rapid development of this new branch of science in Russia. London wrote to Tsar a prophecy: "In coming 20th century power and majesty of the nations will depend on the degree, to which they will acquire the technology of radium". So, the subsequent rapid progress of the USSR in physics and in atomic technologies was not created by Bolshevist government from nowhere: it was based on ideas and deeds of many genius Russian scholars started this process long before Soviet epoch. Russian biomedical science from the late 19th and 20th centuries is world-renowned for its contribution to *neurism*, a doctrine of neural control over body functions in health and disease, first formulated in France by Claude Bernard, but subsequently achieved great results in Russia via efforts of above mentioned I.M. Sechenov, S.P. Botkin, and, of course, Ivan Petrovich Pavlov (1828–1936), the first Russian Nobel Prize winner, and his school.

In neurogerontology significant contribution was given by Russian neurohistologist, multiple nominee for Nobel Prize, A.S. Dogel (1852–1922). This scientist stated that with aging regulatory potential of vegetative nervous system gets weaker, which, in his opinion, may explain the derangement of senile body function and metabolism (Dogel, 1922). Although Maria Kapitonovna Petrova (1874–1948), the closest disciple and dearest co-worker of I.P. Pavlov, attempted to collect experimental and clinical witnesses for cerebral cortex is a key link of senescence (and even has demonstrated that chronic neural stress in dogs causes some acceleration of aging) (Petrova, 1946), neurism, in general, failed to prove that it is the brain which accounts for the weak link of senescence. Moreover, Pavlov himself, unlike some of his followers, underlined the plasticity of CNS and ability of human brain to function perfectly even in very old ages. He proved this with his own long creative life. So, the weak link could be cerebral blood vessels, as mesenchymal structures, but not the brain itself. This was emphasized by pupils of Pavlov and Bogomolets in their "*Manual in Gerontology*", a most fundamental book in world literature of that period (Nagornyi *et al.*, 1963). This seeming failure of neurism in direct assault of the aging problem is not occasional. The neurotransmitters and reflex signals, as a rule, do not regulate cell growth, proliferation and metabolism directly, but intermediate their influence via neuroendocrine or neuroimmune interfaces. That's why Russian neurogeronologists shifted the accents in this field to endocrine facet of a problem. Even the neurovegetative theory of aging, given by Dogel, must be understood in context of central role of hypothalamus as supreme neuroendocrine regulator. Just we need to remember that Dogel wrote within the terms and using the language of his time. In that period hormone–producing activities of hypothalamus were still obscure, so Dogel characterized it as portion of intermediate brain only. To our opinion, in spite of all this limitations of neuristic doctrine, it was mighty enough to contribute significantly into some aspects of gerontology and, first of all, into applied geriatrics. The most valuable result, achieved by this doctrine in Soviet gerontology, probably was derived from research of prominent clinician, founder of Leningrad school of internists: Georgiy Feodorovich Lang (1875–1948) (Fig. 6.15). This physician was the pioneer in formulation of the concepts for two most important diseases of modern elderly people: metabolic syndrome and, especially, hypertonic disease, which term and idea was coined by him (Lang, 1922; 1950). In Western countries, the first description of metabolic syndrome is related to Swedish physician Eskil Kylin (Kylin, 1923), but Lang has noticed and published regular co-morbidity of diabetes mellitus, arterial hypertension, atherosclerosis, obesity and disorders of purine metabolism in elderly patients as early as in 1922. Earlier authors interpreted arterial hypertension as a syndrome caused by various reasons in different patients. Lang was the first who suggested the existence of separate nosological form, brought in by primary disorder in regulation of arterial blood pressure. Moreover, on the basis of neurism he has formulated neurogenic theory of pathogenesis for essential arterial hypertension. WHO, in the beginning of the sixties, characterized

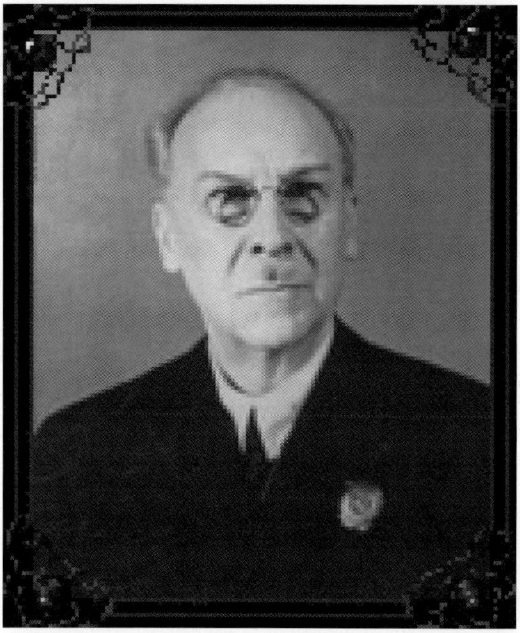

Figure 6.15. Georgiy Feodorovich Lang.

"hypertonic disease" of Lang's book (Lang, 1950) and "essential hypertension" of Western classifications as synonyms, but, in fact this was not correct. The meaning of Lang's term is much broader and deeper, than just simplified statement of primary character of the illness. A typical patient with hypertonic disease initially has essential hypertension, but later on, with aggravation and age progressing of the disease he/she acquires one by one some secondary components of pathogenesis (renal, vascular, cerebral ones etc) in addition to the primary essential one. It means that, according to Lang, advanced hypertonic disease is NOT ONLY essential. These results of Lang's studies are interesting even now, especially for geriatrics, when dealing with advanced cases of hypertension, and are not disputed, even with current predominance of genetic theory in understanding of arterial hypertension.

Another trend of domestic neurogerontology is tightly related to neural control of immune response and neuroimmunological aspects of senility. Two Russian pathophysiologists, Ivan Grigor'evich Savchenko (Savchenko, 1891) and Ye. S. London (London, 1898) — the latter already credited above for his discovery of physiological autoimmunity and origination of Radiobiology — have both demonstrated that some damages of brain may alter significantly the anti-infectious immunity in experimental doves. In continuation, a pupil of Mechnikov and Pavlov, Sergei Ivanovich Metalnikov (1870–1946), a graduate of St. Petersburg University, has conducted in 1926 (together with V.A. Chorine) pioneering experiments in neural regulation of immune response, thus founding the branch of neuroimmunology (Metalnikov and Chorine, 1926). Metalnikov (Fig. 6.16) a protozoologist, studied the aging of unicellular organisms in culture; hence the idea of protozoan "immortality" greatly influenced him. He developed an original neuroimmune gerontological doctrine (Metalnikov, 1917), according which human senescence is not naturally programmed within the cells, but rather interpreted as a result of cumulative effect of

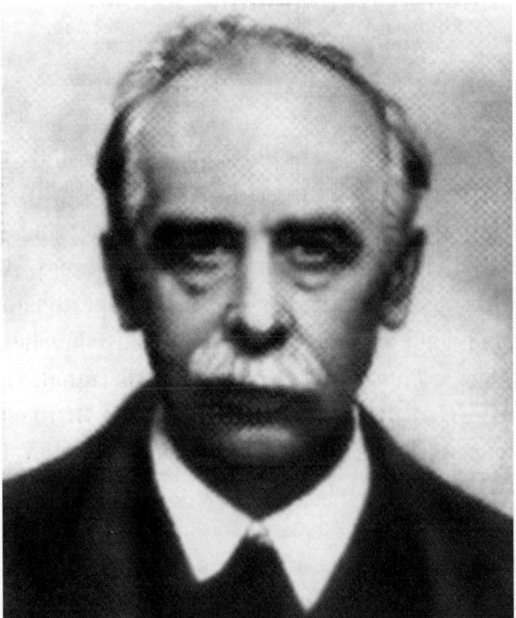

Figure 6.16. Sergei Ivanovich Metal'nikov.

occasional ontogenetic events, damaging the neural control over body functions, including immunity. He produced experimentally anti-cardiac and anti-testicular autoantibodies, causing damage and atrophy of target organs and hypothesized that neuroimmune disorders may result in senility-promoting effects of poorly controlled autoimmunity.

In the beginning of 20th century, with appearance of endocrinology as a branch of Biomedicine, Russian Gerontology developed several interesting endocrinological ideas and theories. Probably one of the earliest domestic endocrinologists (and world protocybernetists) was Nicolay Anatol'evich Belov (1878–1937?) from the same Khar'kov University, which was a real nest of mighty systemic thinkers in Russian Biomedicine. He was the first to coin the idea of servomechanism (negative back circuit) as universal for Physiology and Techniques and illustrated it with some hormonal examples. One of them was the so-called Belov's phenomenon — the experimental decrease of testicle activity in response to delay of prostate gland emptying (Belov, 1911). Belov related this phenomenon to senile decrement of masculine sexual potency. Belov called back circuits "parallel cross-link interactions". Also he postulated that positive back circuits are destructive for complex hierarchical systems, like animal organism, and normally are avoided (Belov, 1911). Later he developed the application of general systems theory to the problem of senescence, insisting that aging phenomena occur, when systemic regulation cumulates failures (Belov, 1924). Belov's precursor in senescence theory was A.A. Bogdanov (see above); much later Belov's idea of destructive positive back circuits will re-incarnate in so called *elevation theory* of senescence (see below). Belov was also the leading Russian adept of physiognomic theory in that period and, like Bogdanov, an active socialist revolutionary.

The practical clinical approach in domestic endocrine gerontology was established by famous pharmacist and chemist from St. Petersburg: Alexander Vasil'evich Poehl (1850–1908). Poehl (Fig. 6.17) owed a very popular drugstore (which still exists at the same place, not far from St. Petersburg University). In late 19th century European scientists were interested in experiments of a French pathophysiologist, Ch.-E. Brown-Sequard (1817–1894), who coined a principle of hormonal regulation. Brown-Sequard at the age of 72 has performed series of experiments on himself, trying to achieve rejuvenation with the help of injections of animal

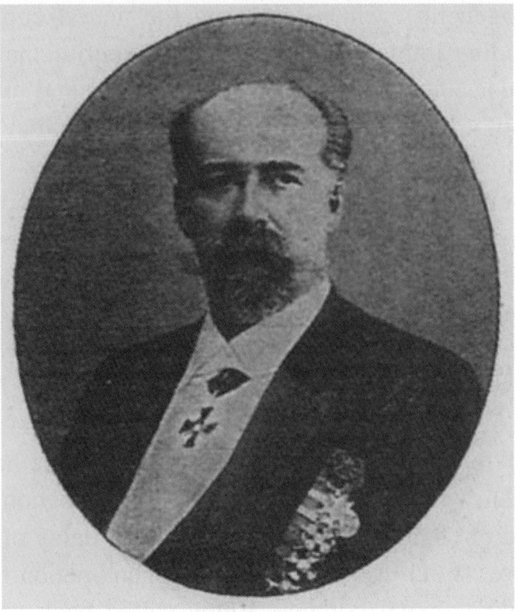

Figure 6.17. Alexander Vasil'evich Poehl.

testicle extract. Poehl has prepared the extract from gonads and semen of animals, purified peptide and polyamine components from it and prescribed these remedies to elderly patients for rejuvenation, sexual stimulation and prevention of senile cardiac diseases. Most popular of these drugs was "*Poehl's spermine*", polyamine purified by Poehl from testicles and semen and proven to be the effective constituent of Brown-Sequard's extracts. Poehl revealed his chemical formula, and correctness of his study was confirmed by D.I. Mendeleev. Due to efforts of A.V. Poehl and I.R. Tarkhnishvili-Tarkhanov (already mentioned above) it has been shown that spermine can stimulate wound healing, Poehl also demonstrated its effect on tissue oxidation and hypothesized that spermine may increase the resistance to Mechnikov's key factor of senility — autointoxication. Now spermine is well-known as anti-inflammatory and reparative autacoid (Zaichik and Churilov, 2008). Recently, a century after Poehl, spermine also was proven to modulate calcium sensor dependant regulation in cardiac muscle (Wang *et al.*, 2003), which re-emphasizes the principal correctness of Poehl's approach.

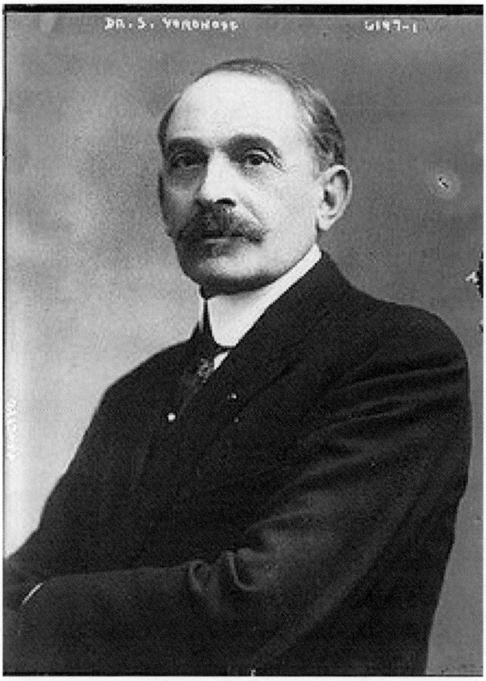

Figure 6.18. Serge (Samuel) Abramovich Voronov.

Poehl's doctrine of treatment with extracts of animal organs called "opotherapy" had considerable impact on medical community in Russia, especially as regards to geriatrics (Poehl, 1903).

This approach has been developed farther by prominent Russian-French experimental gerontologist and geriatric surgeon Serge (Samuel) Abramovich Voronov (1866–1951). Voronov (Fig. 6.18) was influenced by the works of Alexis Carrel (1873–1944), the youngest Nobel Prize winner of that time (a French-American experimental surgeon and explorer of cell immortality in culture). Also he took some experience from his medical practice in Middle East, where he has noticed signs of early senility in eunuchs. Voronov decided to prevent or even reverse aging effects by means of xenogenic grafting of gonads from monkey to human (Voronoff, 1926). After series of experiments on animals first successful graft of testicular tissue from chimpanzee and baboon monkey to man was made by Voronov on June 12th, 1920. In twenties, this method of experimental treatment brought him world fame and lot of prosperous elderly patients. Later, with discovery of testosterone and recognition of graft rejection, Voronov's approach was abandoned, but many modern analysts advocate him and credit for his early promotion of the trend, which went later to the studies of Swiss doctor Paul Niehans (1882–1971), who has rejuvenated the celebrities with prototype cellular therapy. Next steps of this pathway lead to modern stem cell therapy, used now broadly for treatment of senile cell-deficient diseases.

In the late 19th and early 20th centuries endocrine physiologists stood very close to discovery of the thyroid hormones. It was already clear due to efforts of Germans Max Rubner (see above) and Adolf Magnus-Levy (1865–1955), that thyroid gland incretion is able to regulate the level of oxidative metabolism and resting metabolic rate of the body. Taken together with the above-mentioned Rubner's theory, which insisted that longevity depends on total energy expenditure and senescence is a function of the metabolic speed (Sinclair and Guarente, 2006), these facts pushed gerontologists to the search of thyroid reasons for aging. As early as in 1891 Scottish physician George Redmayne Murray (1865–1939) successfully treated severe myxoedema in an almost dying senile 46-year-old lady-patient by means of organotherapy with the hypodermic injections of sheep's thyroid extract. Doctor supported her on this treatment for 28 years. A similar method of treatment for goiter and even for related cretinism was used long ago by ancient Chinese physician Sūn Sīmiǎo (581–682), but it was not known in Europe before Murray (Slater, 2010). In 1910 an Austrian health resort physician Arnold Lorand (Fig. 6.23) from Karlovy Vary has related senescence to hypothyroidism, noticed similarity in their manifestation and suggested that thyroid hormones are geroprotectors. He wrote: "We can produce experimentally typical symptoms of old age in young animals by extirpation of the ductless glands, more especially the thyroid…" (Lorand, 2003). In Russia similar ideas were proclaimed by an outstanding endocrinologist Nikolay Adolphovich Shereshevskiy (1885–1961) (Fig. 6.19). This physician was the first (1925) who described a classical phenotype of a chromosomal disease manifested in congenital primary ovarian failure, now known in English-speaking countries as Turner's syndrome (1938) and called in Russia Shereshevskiy-Turner' syndrome. This syndrome is

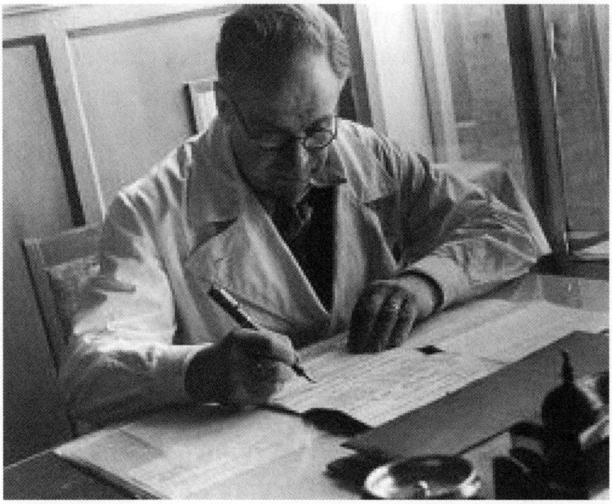

Figure 6.19. The pioneer of hypothyroid theory of premature senescence in Russia: Nicolay Adolphovich Shereshevskiy.

characterized by a very high incidence of autoimmune thyroiditis (AIT) in patients. AIT is progressive chronic disease causing hypothyroidism, which accelerates senescence and age-related diseases, like atherosclerosis and metabolic syndrome (see below). That's why Shereshevskiy, who studied these patients for a long time, could not miss the early senility in them. As a result, he insisted on hypothyroidism and hypogonadism to be the main mechanisms of senescence (Shereshevskiy, 1940). Shereshevskiy later headed the first Soviet Research Institute of Endocrinology and Hormone Chemistry (1934–1953) and collaborated at Kremlin's hospital for Soviet leaders, whose cheerfulness he supported by means of endocrinological treatment. In 1953 during campaign of mass repressions against Kremlin physicians he was arrested and accused to be "foreign spy". He was liberated from prison after Stalin's death, as well as A.L. Chizhevskiy, mentioned above. But many talented Russian thinkers perished in that period, like N.A. Belov, for whom even date of death is not known exactly.

We need to make here an excursion into organizational history of Soviet gerontology and geriatrics. The Soviet model of socialism not only established (for the first time in domestic history) a variety of social guarantees and benefits for elderly people. To a certain degree, the whole social system, step by step, acquired definite *gerontocratic* accent. The Great October revolution of 1917 was an uprising, which brought to power very young politicians. Vladimir Il'ich Lenin in his 47 was eldest among all members of first Soviet government (so-called Soviet of People's Commissars). All others were much younger (excerpt I.I. Skvortsov-Stepanov, People's Commissar of Finances, close friend of gerontologist Bogdanov, also 47 years old to that moment). But, because of conservative and rigid social structure of later Soviet state, those in power were getting older and older. At least, the average age of leaders had increased with every decade. It looks quite natural that these leaders pay enough attention to progress in life prolongation and advances of geriatric medicine. Gerontology and geriatrics in the USSR were always in the scope of state care. Both research and health care measures in this field were properly financed. As early as in 1938 in Kiev through the initiative of Mechnikov's disciple and Bogdanov's co-worker A.A. Bogomolets, who was widely supported by state, the first research conference in Gerontology and Geriatrics was organized, the earliest symposium of this type in the history of world science. The largest and most fruitful academic school of gerontologists was formed in Soviet Ukraine, at Kiev — around A.A. Bogomolets; and at Khar'kov, around Alexandr Vasil'evich Nagornyi (1887–1953), well-known gerontophysiologist and gerontobiochemist (Nagornyi, 1963). The first local gerontological societies were established in 1957 at Leningrad and, a few months later, at Moscow. In 1958 the Soviet Academy of Sciences opened its first Research Institute of Gerontology in Kiev. In 1963 (also in Kiev) the first all-union Congress in Gerontology and Geriatrics proclaimed the foundation of the Soviet Research and Medical Society of Gerontologists and Geriatrists. It functioned until the split of the USSR, then the first international gerontological symposium in the USSR (1967) as well as the 9th World Congress in Gerontology (1972) were organized. The first teaching Department of Gerontology and Geriatrics for postgraduate training was established in our country in 1970 (at Kiev). In the last decade of Soviet history (1978–1990), a broad and ambitious complex state program for development of gerontology and geriatrics was realized in the USSR (with involvement of 39 universities and research institutes); this led to the creation of a specialized geriatric service within the public health system and the establishment of a periodic national specialized academic journal: "*Problems of Aging and Longevity*" — published quarterly since 1990. But, after the split of the country, a considerable part of this Soviet heritage stayed beyond the borders of post-Soviet Russia, and many national links of this system (research society, national peer-reviewed journal, academic council etc.) have to be re-established. Currently two domestic research institutions function in our country: St. Petersburg Research Institute of Bioregulation and Gerontology (1992) and Moscow Research Institute of Gerontology (1997). Postgraduate training in this field is established at Departments of Gerontology and Geriatrics of Moscow Medical Academy of Postgraduate Studies and I.I. Mechnikov North-West Medical University of St. Petersburg. Samara Medical University and I.M. Sechenov 1st Moscow Medical University — both have Departments of Gerontology and Geriatrics for the training of graduate students. This data and current situation in domestic gerontology and in geriatric social and health care are discussed in monograph by V.N. Anisimov (2003), as well as in our recent publications (Stroev *et al.*, 2009; 2010).

It is not surprising that Soviet scientists were quite active in the area of gerontology and geriatrics and have achieved many interesting results (Duplenko, 2012). Besides the achievements already described earlier, we shall mention several comprehensive manuals in this field, written by leading specialists, broadly published in the USSR and influenced the research interests of many young scientists. Among those first Soviet monographs on this matter, some already quoted above: by A.V. Nagornyi (1923), M.S. Müehlman (1927), A.A. Bogomolets (1940), and especially the fundamental volume by A.V. Nagornyi *et al.* (1963). A very bright monograph in Gerontology was authored by great Soviet pathologist Hippolyte Vasil'evich Davydovskiy (1887–1968) (Davydovskiy, 1966), and later, considerable contributions in this area were represented in an academic manual in mechanisms of aging edited by V.V Frol'kis *et al.* (1982), and a practical manual in Geriatrics edited by D.F. Chebotariov (1982). Perhaps the last top achievements of gerontology in Soviet period were related to the names of two outstanding domestic scientists: Vladimir Mikhailovich Dil'man (1925–1994) (Fig. 6.20) and Alexey Matveevich Olovnikov (born 1936) (Fig. 6.21).

Dil'man (1971) has formulated an original *"elevation theory"* of aging. According this concept, senescence is indirect, side effect of realization of certain genetic programs related to metabolic regulation. Hypothalamus, which is major regulator of balance constants in our body, supreme link

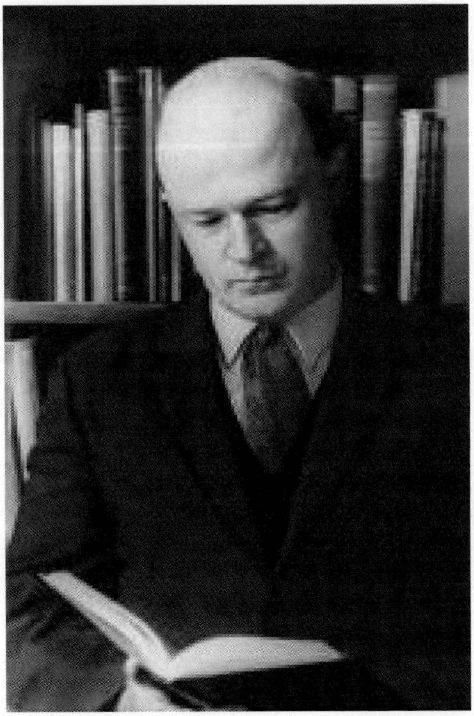

Figure 6.20. Vladimir Mikhailovich Dil'man, author of elevation theory.

of neuroendocrine interface and affective conductor of human behavior, is sensitive to many physiological and metabolic parameters (body temperature, body mass, osseous mass, arterial blood pressure, extracellular fluid tonicity, blood levels of many hormones and metabolites) (Zaichik and Churilov, 2008). The decline or elevation of these parameters is compensated by hypothalamus via endocrine and/or autonomous nervous systems. Dil'man coined in an idea that the thresholds of sensitivity for hypothalamic sensors, controlling these parameters, tend to elevate with aging. This results in shift of many metabolic and physiological parameters in senile organism towards higher ranges (including blood pressure, cholesterol and glucose levels, body mass, levels of stress hormones and growth hormone/insulin-like growth factor 1, etc). According elevation theory, this mechanism is responsible for metabolic syndrome, decrease of reproductive potential and increase of stress-related changes ("*hyperadaptosis*")

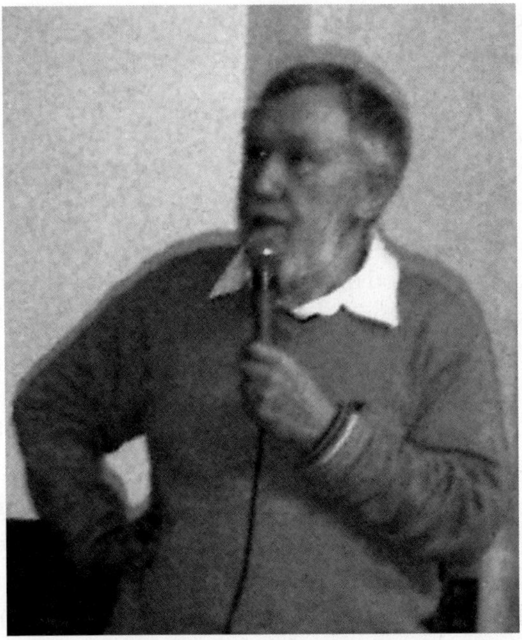

Figure 6.21. Alexey Matveevich Olovnikov, originator of telomere hypothesis.

in aged persons. The change of metabolic situation, in turn, facilitates the pathogenesis of cellular immunity decline and promotes tumor growth, cardiovascular and stress-related diseases of senility. Dil'man's school has collected many experimental and clinical epidemiological witnesses for this theory (Dil'man, 1971; 1978; 1981; 1987; 1994).

Alexey Matveevich Olovnikov (Fig. 6.21) is a leading Russian theoretician in the field of Systemic Biology, who has coined in an idea of "*marginotomy*" (1971). According his theory, "*the incomplete copying of template margin in enzymatic synthesis of polynucleotides*" is of crucial biological significance in the phenomenon of cell senescence and can explain the "Heyflick's limit" for a number of generations in cell cultures. As a result of DNA polymerase inability to copy entire length of a template, with every new cell division a replica gets shorter and shorter. A cell lifespan is countered by this mechanism (Olonikov, 1973). Olovnikov remembered that the idea came to him while he was watching a train in suburbs of Moscow, which stopped by a platform, being some shorter in length. Fourteen years later this brilliant Olovnikov's guess came true, and telomerase was discovered by C.W. Greinder and E.H. Blackburn (1985) as an enzyme able to re-elongate telomeres in immortal neoplastic, stem and protozoan cells. Although the discoverers repeatedly referred to Olovnikov's paper, which was translated into English in 1973 (Olonikov, 1973) and broadly known to Western researchers, the Nobel committee has omitted the name of the theory originator when it awarded this trend of studies with the Nobel Prize in 2009, and we do not know any reason. This decision was not understood or approved by perplexed Russian gerontological community. In 2009 Russians awarded Olovnikov with Demidov Prize (named after famous domestic industrial magnate, analogue of Nobel), symbolically correcting the decision of Nobel committee (Yegorov and Zelenin, 2011). Regardless of recognition matters, A.M. Olovnikov made a new important step in his theoretical search and constructed in 2003 an elegant hypothesis, trying to combine telomerase mechanism of cellular aging and Dil'man's elevation theory of senescence with some data on the role of insulin resistance in systemic aging. The aim was to understand the phenomenon of whole body senescence (Olovnikov, 2003). This concept is known as "*chronomere*" theory and, perhaps, represents an attempt of most global synthesis in theoretical Gerontology. According his hypothesis (Olonikov, 2005), small linear perichromosomal DNA molecules, so-called *redusomes*, may function as intranuclear organelles (for example, in hypothalamic cells), and their non-occasional shortening with course of time results in elevation of thresholds of sensitivity for hypothalamic metabolic sensors, thus provoking intermediate brain senescence and systemic aging. A hypothetical mechanism for that is linked by Olovnikov to periodical phenomena, caused by Moon gravitation. This theory definitely is crazy enough to be true! But, in this case, people probably will cease to get old, if they will migrate from the Cradle of Mankind to some other planet, devoid of natural satellites, let say — Venus.

Russian gerontology and geriatrics always were inherent to the endocrine aspects of senescence in the scope of domestic aging studies, and not only thyroid and pituitary, mentioned above. For a long time the main hero of this story use to be the pineal body. French philosopher Rene Descartes (Fig. 6.22) in the 17th century has positioned the immortal sole of human being into this organ. More than 200 years later (in 1958) Soviet endocrine pathologist Arnold M. Helimskiy has demonstrated the fact of its

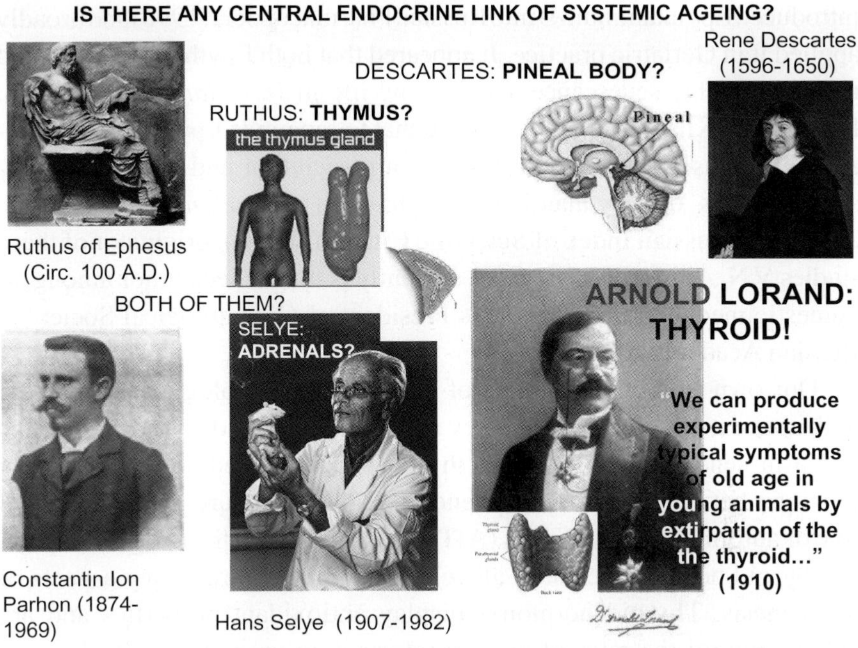

Figure 6.22. Endocrine conceptions of senescence and their authors.

senile involution (Helimskiy, 1958). A bit earlier (1955) his Rumanian colleague Constantin Ion Parhon, a very prolific scientist and public leader who had published the world's first textbook of Endocrinology and was in 1948–1952 the first President of Rumanian Republic, discovered that pineal extracts may cause life prolongation in old rats (Parhon, 1955). Later due to efforts of J. Axelrod and others, melatonin was discovered with photoperiodicity of its incretion, which brought to epiphysis the status of the organism's sun clock (Erren and Reiter, 2010). The pineal peptide extract named "Epytalaminum©" was prepared by Soviet gerontologists V.N. Anisimov, V.Kh. Khavinson, V.G. Morozov and V.M. Dil'man, and proven (1973) to cause life prolongation, anti-oxidative, melatonin-stimulating effects in rats, as well as restore their reproductive ability in old age (Anisimov, 2003; Khavinson *et al.*, 2001). Pineal peptides apparently delayed the senile changes of neuroendocrine regulation involved in elevation mechanism of systemic aging. Later the authors introduced Epytalaminum© into Russian Pharmacopoeia (1990) and broadly applied it in Geriatric practice. It appeared that both Epythalaminum© and melatonin delay senescence and prolong life in *D. melanogaster* (1997). Later V. Kh. Khavinson *et al.*, showed that tetrapeptide Epytalon (Ala-Glu-Asp-Gly) was able to regulate melatonin secretion and reproduce anti-senile effects of Epytalaminum© extract in *D. melanogaster* (2002). According Russian Index of Scientific Citation (RISC), originator of these studies V.N. Anisimov (Fig. 6.23) currently is most cited author among all domestic medical scientists. He is President of Gerontological Society at Russian Academy of Sciences.

Our own studies in the field of endocrine gerontology were inspired with above mentioned ideas on key roles of autoimmunity and connective tissue in senescence, as well as thyroid studies, cited above. We study relations between marfanoid phenotype and premature senescence and role of autoimmune thyroiditis (AIT) for early metabolic aging. Receptors for thyroid hormones exist in all cells, thus they control many aspects of ontogenesis. Thyroid hormones display antioxidant properties and are able to control the rates of genetic information processing (Zaichik and Churilov, 2008; Zaichik *et al.*, 2008). Hence, the thyroid status and anti-thyroid autoimmunity are of great meaning for aging, cell renewal and age-related diseases. Hypothyroidism in non-iodine deficient regions (and

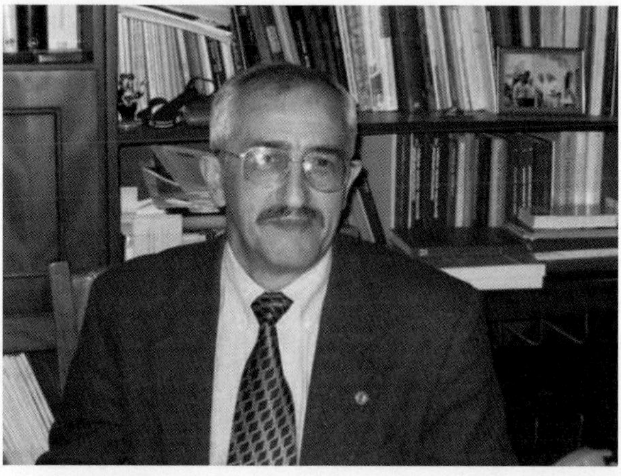

Figure 6.23 Vladimir Nikolaevich Anisimov, at present — leading Russian gerontologist.

among persons older than six) worldwide is caused mainly by Hashimoto's chronic AIT, a social disease, which prevalence among females in some areas is up to 25%, according post-mortem pathomorphological screening, and increases with age (Williams and Doniach, 1962). AIT, even started in adolescence, is a life-long disease, causing accelerated senescence after few decades of its course (geroderma, decrease of mental and physical activity, emotional blunt, hair loss, depression of libido, accelerated atherosclerosis etc.). Our prospective clinical and pathophysiological study of 3000 patients with AIT from adolescent to old age revealed the interaction of hypothyroidism and progressive autoallergy in acceleration of aging (Fig. 6.24) (Churilov *et al.*, 2009). Moreover, it appeared that

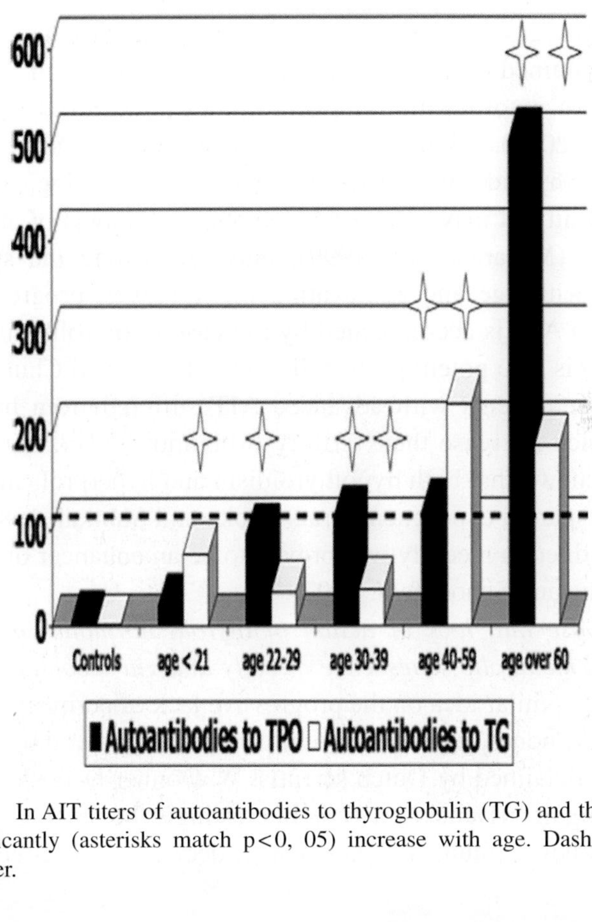

Figure 6.24. In AIT titers of autoantibodies to thyroglobulin (TG) and thyroperoxidase (TPO) significantly (asterisks match p<0, 05) increase with age. Dashed line shows diagnostic titer.

individuals with inherited polygenic multifactorial connective tissue disorders of marfanoid phenotype are predisposed to AIT. In such individuals a highly spread adolescent disorder named hypothalamic syndrome of puberty (also known as Simpson-Page syndrome or juvenile obesity with rose striae) rapidly transgresses into early complicated metabolic syndrome and accelerated senescence with multiorganic autoimmune involvement. The mechanism of this transgression in such individuals is related to chronic systemic excess of TGF-beta, leptin, prolactin and several pro-inlammatory cytokines (Stroev and Churilov, 2011; Stroev *et al.*, 2011). Treatment with thyroid hormones in AIT up till now was regarded as substitutive only. However, autoallergy in AIT is multi-targeted and involves other endocrine and non-endocrine cells as well. Earlier it has been shown that thyroid hormones in experiment inhibit the development of autoimmune gastritis (Wang *et al.*, 1998). Hypothyroidism is known to retard programmed cell death (Zaichik *et al.*, 2008; Singh *et al.*, 2003). Withdrawal of autoimmune lymphoid clones is achieved via apoptosis (Coico *et al.*, 2005). Taking all this into account, we suggested that growing deficit of thyroid hormones in AIT alters the physiological regulation of autoimmunity. It may delay the apoptotic withdrawal of auto-reactive lymphocytes (Mihara *et al.*, 1999), thus broadening the spectrum of autoallergy with age and aggravating it. Moreover, progressive hypothyroidism in AIT is accompanied by increase in thyroliberin secretion. Thyroliberin is also potent prolactoliberin (Zaichik and Churilov, 2008), hence all our patients with advanced AIT suffered from hyperprolactinemia, which decrease their fertility (Maximova *et al.*, 2011). Earlier it has been shown that both hypothyroidism and hyperprolactinemia may alter the lifespan in experimental rats (Ooka and Shinkai, 1986). Finally, hyperprolactinemia recently was proven to be an enhancer of autoimmunity (Orbacha and Schoenfeld, 2007).

We suppose that lack of action of thyroid hormones may promote immune and metabolic senescence directly and via secondary hyperprolactinemia. A similar idea on the progressive lack of peripheral sensitivity to thyroid hormones, especially within immune and cardiovascular systems, was proclaimed by Dutch scientist W. Donner Denckla as a reason for aging long ago (Denckla, 1974). Interestingly, he related that to effect of some unknown pituitary factor, which decreases the effectiveness of thyroid regulation with age (so-called "death hormone") (Denckla, 1975). In our opinion, this hypothetical factor may be associated to prolactin regulation. Based on these findings and on above listed assumptions, we have suggested (Churilov *et al.*, 2009) a new therapeutic method for multi-organic autoallergy and premature senility, and treated 77 patients (25-67 years) with multi-organic autoallergy (combined autoimmune: thyroiditis, thrombocytopenia, adrenalitis, gastritis with megaloblastic anemia, insulin-dependant diabetes mellitus and rheumatoid arthritis). All patients were previously unsuccessfully treated with glucocorticoids. In one case (with severe autoimmune thrombocytopenia) splenectomy was even performed, but without effect. In spite of standard prolonged immunosuppressive treatment with glucocorticoids the number of platelets remained critically low; sometimes falling down to 10×10^9/L. Levels of antithyroid autoantibodies in these patients were inversely related to blood plasma cortisol and directly related to prolactin levels (Maximova *et al.*, 2011). Because all patients had clinical and laboratory manifestations of hypothyroidism, we have administered them course of L-thyroxine©. In all patients this resulted in normalization of blood platelet count; in three of them total withdrawal of glucocorticoids became possible, and all others have successfully reduced their Prednisolone© doasage. This can not be explained with stimulation of thrombopoiesis, because thyroid hormones are known to lower it (Cordiano *et al.*, 1998). We suggest that thyroid hormones accelerate the apoptosis of autoreactive lymphoid clones, thus suppressing the autoallergic thrombocytolysis. Significant decrease in titers of anti-platelet autoantibodies and increase in platelet number were paralleled with visual signs of "rejuvenation" due to disappearance of geroderma and myxoedema in patient. Prolactin level in patients after treatment with thyroid hormones decreased, because of achieved euthyroidism and diminished thyroliberin production (Fig. 6.25).

Hence, application of thyroid hormones in AIT produces not only substitutive, but immune modulating effect, because it suppresses immunopathogenic hyperprolactinemia. The curative potential of L-thyroxine© in age-related autoallergic disorders should be re-estimated and, in our opinion, it can rival glucocorticoids with the advantage of the absence of adverse effects, which are particularly undesirable for old people and typical for glucocorticoid treatment. Recently it has been shown that

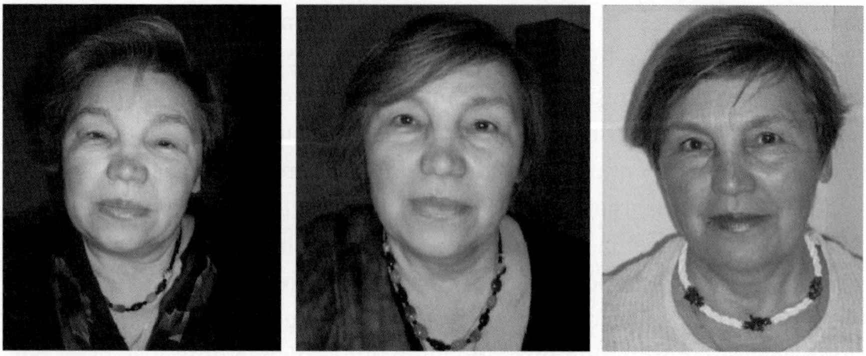

Figure 6.25. Reverse dynamics of accelerated aging after cure of multi-organic autoallergy with L-thyroxine©. Patient P.N., 59 years; case history No 112; *Left*: 18.01. 07 before (blood TSH = 200 mcU/ml, T3 = 0,0 nM/l); *Middle*: 18.03.07, during course of treatment; *Right*: 04.06.07 — after treatment (TSH = 54 mcU/ml; T3 = 1, 18 nM/l).

prolonged administration of L-thyroxine© is able to stimulate human sirtuin-1 expression (Engel and Mahlknecht, 2008). Taken together, all this data may suggest that prevention and appropriate treatment of AIT may serve as an important method of prophylaxis for premature senility and early metabolic syndrome, especially among persons with marfanoid phenotype.

References

Anisimov, V.N. (2003) *Molecular and Physiological Mechanisms of Aging*. Nauka Publishing, St. Petersburg.

Belov, N.A. (1911) Doctrine of inner secretion of organs and tissues and its meaning in modern medicine. *Novoe v Meditsine* **22**, 1228–1236.

Belov, N.A. (1924) Physiology of types. In: *An Experience of Research in Psycho-Physical Characteristics of Personality Depending on Ergonomogenesis*. Krasnaya Kniga Publishing, Oryol.

Bergonier, J. and Tribondeau, L. (1905) Actions des rayons X sur le testicule du rat blanc. C. r. Seanc. *Soc. Biol.* **58**, 154–158, 678–680.

Bogdanoff, A.A. (1927) Zur Theorie des Alterns. *Russische-Deutsch. Med. Zeitschrift.* **1**, 3–17.

Bogdanov, A.A. (1980) Essays in tektology. In: *The General Science of Organization*. (Translator Gorelik, G.) Intersystems Publishing Ltd., Seaside, California.

Bogdanov, A.A. (2002) In: *The Struggle for Viability: Collectivism through Blood Exchange* (Translator, ed.) Huestis, D. W. Xlibris, Philadelphia.

Bogomolets, A.A. (1909) On the physiology of adrenal glands. Suprarenotoxins. *Russ. vrach.* **29**, 972–978.

Bogomolets, A.A. (1940) *The Life Prolongation. Acad. Sci.* Ukr. SSR Publishing, Kyiv.

Chebotariov, D.F. and Man'kovskiy, N.B. (eds.) *Manual in Geriatrics*. Meditsina Publishing, Moscow, 1982.

Chizhevsky, A.L. (1976) *The Terrestrial Echo of Solar Storms*. Progress Publishing, Moscow.

Churilov, L.P. and Shmeliov, A.A. (2008) Under the "Rose and Cross" sign. In search for panacea in Russia. *Meditsina — XXI vek.* **3**(12), 70–83.

Churilov, L.P., Stroev, Yu.I. and Mudzhikova, O.M. (2009) Ageing, thyroid and autoallergy: new insight into pathogenesis and treatment. *Wien. Klin. Wochenschr.* **121**(7–8), 70–71.

Churilov, L.P., Stroev, Yu.I. and Utekhin, V.J., *et al.* (2010) Science of body imperfection: from pathophysiology to pathobiology via innovative interdisciplinary teaching. In: *The 6th International Congress of Pathophysiology — 14th International SHR Symposium on Gene-Environment Interaction in Health and Disease*, Sept. 22nd–25th, 2010, Montreal, Canada. ISP Publishing, Montreal, pp. 29.

Coico, R., Sunshine, G. and Benjamini, E. (2005) *Immunology: A Short Course*, 5th ed. Wiley, Hoboken.

Cordiano, I., Betterle, C. and Spadaccino, C.A., *et al.* (1998) Autoimmune thrombocytopenia (AITP) and thyroid autoimmune disease (TAD), overlapping syndromes? *Clin. Exptl. Immunol.* **113**, 373–378.

Davydovskiy, H.V. (1966) *Gerontology*. Meditsina Publishing, Moscow.

Denckla, D.W. (1974) Role of the pituitary and thyroid glands in the decline of minimal O_2 consumption with age. *J. Clin. Invest.* **53**, 572–581.

Denckla, D.W. (1975) A time to die. *Life Sci.* **16**(1), 31–44.

Dilman, V.M. (1971) Age-associated elevation of hypothalamic threshold to feedback control and its role in development, aging and disease. *Lancet* **1**, 1211–1219.

Dilman, V.M. (1978) Aging, metabolic immunodepression and carcinogenesis. *Mech. Ageing Dev.* **8**, 153–173.

Dilman, V.M. (1981) *The Law of Deviation of Homeostasis and Diseases of Aging.* J. Wright PSG Ltd., Boston.

Dil'man, V.M. (1987) *Four Models of Medicine*. Meditsina Publishing, Moscow.

Dilman, V.M. (1994) *Development, Aging and Disease. A New Rationale for an Intervention Strategy* (Translator Young, J.K.). Harwood Academic Publishing, Chur, Switzerland.

Dogel, A.S. (1922) *Old Age and Death*. Mysl' Publishing, Petrograd.

Dontsov, V.I. (1998) The lymphocyte-mediated regulation of cell growth in somatic tissues and new immune theory of senescence. *Profilaktika Starenija* **1**, 40–63. Available from: http://medi.ru/doc/708013.htm

Duplenko, Y.K. (2012) Academic relations in gerontology. In: *Science and Technics: Problems of History and Theory*, Issue 28. SPbFNIIET RAN Publisher, St. Petersburg, pp. 154–155.

Emanuel, N.M. (1985) Kinetics and free-radical mechanisms of ageing and carcinogenesis. In: *Age-Related Factors in Carcinogenesis* (eds.) Likhachev, A.J., Anisimov, V.N. and Montesano, R. IARC Science Publishing, Lyon, pp. 127–149.

Engel, N. and Mahlknecht, U. (2008) Aging and anti-aging: unexpected side effects of everyday medication through sirtuin1 modulation. *Int. J. Molec. Med.* **21**(2), 223–232.

Erren, T.C. and Reiter, R.J. (2010) Axelrod, the pineal and the melatonin hypothesis: lessons of 50 years to shape chronodisruption research. *Neuro. Endocrinol Lett.* **31**(5), 585–587.

Feodorov, N.F. (1982) *Compositions*. Mysl' Publishing, Moscow.

Fischer, J.B. (1760) De senio eiusque gradibus et morbis nec non de eiusdem acquisitione tractatus: accesserunt praeterae Franc. Ranchini, et Floyeri Gerocomicarum amplae sciagraphiae; nec non Welstedii et Dethardingii Conspirante quasi longaevitatem fato... Officina Weberiana, Erfurt, pp. 324.

Frol'kis, V.V. (1982) *Biology of Senescence*, Manual in Physiology series (eds.) Frol'kis, V.V., *et al.* Nauka Publishing, Leningrad.

Greider, C.W. and Blackburn, E.H. (1985) Identification of a specific telomere terminal transferase activity in *Tetrahymena* extracts. *Cell* **51**, 405–413.

Gruman, G.J. (1966) A history of ideas about the prolongation of life. *Transact. Am. Philos. Soc.* **56**, 3–102.

Gumilev, L.N. (1990) *Ethnogenesis and Biosphere*. Progress Publishing, Moscow.

Harman, D. (1956) Aging: a theory based on free radical and radiation chemistry. *J. Gerontol.* **11**, 298–300.

Helimskiy, A.M. (1958) To the question of age changes in pineal gland. *Probl. Endocrinol.* **4**(2), 96–100.

Huestis, D.W. (2007) Alexander Bogdanov: the forgotten pioneer of blood transfusion. *Transfus. Med. Rev.* **21**, 337–340.

Kad'jan, A.A. (1890) *The Population of St. Petersburg Municipal Hospices (The Materials for Studies of Senility According to Research of 1889 Supervised by S.P. Botkin).* Schreder's Publishing, St. Petersburg.

Kay, M.M.B. (1983) Appearance of a terminal differentiation antigen on senescent and damaged cells and its implications for physiologic autoantibodies. *Biomembranes* **11**, 119–156.

Khavinson, V.Kh., Morozov, V.C. and Anisimov, V.N. (2001) Experimental studies of the pineal gland preparation epithalamin. In: *The Pineal Gland and Cancer. Neuroimmunoendocrine Mechanisms in Malignancy* (eds.) Bartsch, C., Bartsch, H., Blask, D.E., *et al.* Springer Verlag, Berlin, pp. 294–306.

Khavinson, V.Kh. (2002) Peptides and ageing. *Neuroendocrinol. Lett.* **23**(Suppl 3), 1–144.

Kylin, E. (1923) Studien ueber das hypertonie-hyperglykamie-hyperurikamie syndrom. *Zentralbl. f. Inn. Med.* **44**, 105–127.

Lang, G.F. (1922) About hypertonia. *Arch. Gos. Klin. Inst. Usoversh. Vrachej (Leningrad).* **I**, 16–66.

Lang, G.F. (1950) *The Hypertonic Disease*. Medgiz Publishing, Leningrad.

Lomonosov, M.V. (1950) *Selected Philosophical Works.* Gospolitizdat Publishing, Moscow, pp. 598–614.

London, Ye.S. (1899) About the influence of removal of various cerebral parts on immunity towards anthrax. *Arch. Biol. Nauk.* **7**, 177–187.

London, Ye.S. (1901) On the doctrine of spermolysins. *Arkh. Biol. Nauk.* **9**(1), 82–127.

London, E.S. (1911) *Das Radium in der Biologie und Medizin*. Akadem. Verlags., Leipzig, pp. 199.

Lorand, A. (2003) *Old Age Deferred*, 5th Ed. Kessinger Publishing, Whitefish, MT, p. 532.

Lumière, A. (1921) Rôle des Colloïdes chez les Etres Vivants. Essai de Biocollodologie; Nouvelles Hypothèses dans le Domaine de la Biologie, et de la Médicine. Masson et Cie, Paris.

Malinovskiy, A.A. (1986) Senility from the Evolutionist's Point of View. *Priroda* **8**, 81–89.

Marinesco, G. (1928) Nouvelles recherches sur les plaques seniles. *L'Encuphale* **23**, 697.

Maximova, A.V., Pinigina, Yu.I., Stroev, Yu.I., Zhao, W., Churilov, L.P. (2011) Hashimoto's autoimmune thyroiditis, hypothyroidism, prolactin and female reproductive system. *Actual. Probl. Transp. Med.* **2**(24), 122–130.

Metalnikov, S.I. (1917) *Problem of Immortality in Modern Biology*. Kuhelhen, Glitch and Co., Petrograd, p. 64.

Metalnikov, S. and Chorine, V.A. (1926) Role des reflexes conditionnels dans l'immunite. *Ann. de L'Instit. Pasteur* **11**, 893.

Metchnikoff, E. (1892) In: *The Evolutionary Biology Papers of Elie Metchnikoff* (eds.) Gourko, H., Williamson, D.I. and Tauber, A.I. Kluwer Acad. Publishing, Dordrecht, 2000, pp. 207–216.

Metchnikoff, E.I. (1901) Cell poisons and cytotoxins. *Russkij Arkh. Patol., Klin. Med. i Bakteriol.* **11**(2), 101.

Metchnikoff, E.I. (1902) Alexandr Onufrievich Kovalevskiy. *Vestnik Evropy* **6**(12), 772–799.

Metchnikoff, E. (1903) *The Nature of Man. Studies in Optimistic Philosophy* (Translator Mitchell, P.Ch.). W. Heinemann Publishing, London, p. 328.

Metchnikoff, E. and Rue, E. (1914) L'oeuvre de Paul Ehrlich. *Berliner Klin. Wschr.* **1**, 523–531.

Müehlman, M.S. (1927) The doctrine of growth, senescence and death. Baku, 1926. German version: Mühlmann M. Wachstum, Altern und Tod. Ober die Ursache des Alterns und des Todes. *Ergeb. Anat. Entw. Gesch.* **27**, 1–245.

Nagornyi, A.V. (1923) *The Life, Old Age and Death*. Gosizdat Ukrajiny Publishing, Odessa, p. 120.

Nagornyi, A.V., Nikitin, V.N. and Bulankin, I.N. (1963) *Problem of Senescence and Longevity*. Medgiz Publishing, Moscow.

Odin, V.I., Bogdanov, A.N. and Tsygan, V.N. *et al.* (2008) S.P. Botkin as the founder of home clinical gerontology. *Adv. Gerontol.* **21**(2), 177–180.

Olovnikov, A.M. (1971) Principle of marginotomy in template synthesis of polynucleotides. *Dokl. Akad. Nauk. SSSR* **201**, 1496–1499.

Olovnikov, A.M. (1973) A theory of marginotomy. The incomplete copying of template margin in enzymic synthesis of polynucleotides and biological significance of the phenomenon. *J. Theor. Biol.* **41**(1), 181–190.

Olovnikov, A.M. (2003) Redusome hypothesis of aging and control of biological time in ontogeny. *Biochemistry* (*Moscow*) **68**, 2–33.

Olovnikov, A.M. (2005) Primary cause of aging is in shortening of redumeres — perichromosomal linear DNA molecules, but completely not telomeres — rulers of biological time. *Phenomenon and noumenon of Time*. **2**(2), 294–316. Available from: http://www.chronos.msu.ru/journal/files/archive/2005/02/11_olovnikov_pervoprichina.pdf

Ooka, H. and Shinkai, T. (1986) Effects of chronic hyperthyroidism on the lifespan of the rats. *Mech. Ageing Dev.* **33**, 275–282.

Orbacha, H. and Schoenfeld, Y. (2007) Hyperprolactinemia and autoimmune diseases. *Autoimmun. Rev.* **6**(8), 537–542.

Osborn, T.B., Mendel, L.B., Ferry, I.L., *et al.* (1917) The effect of retardation of growth upon the breeding period and duration of the life in rats. *Science* **45**, 294–295.

Parhon, C.I. (1955) *Biologia Virstelor; Cercetari Clinice si Experimentale*. Editura Acad. Rep. Popul. Romine, Buchureşt, p. 451

Perelman, L.R. (1966) The doctrine of cytotoxins. In: *Manual in Pathological Physiology*. V.I. Meditsina Publishing, Moscow, pp. 430–449.

Petrova, M.K. (1946) *On the Role of Functionally Weakened Cerebral Cortex in Origin of Different Pathological Processes in Organism*. Medgiz Publishing, Leningrad, p. 95.

Pictét, A. (1916) Structure of molecules and life. *Priroda* **4**(4), 421–436.

Pirogov, N.I. (2008) *The Questions of Life. Dairy of an Old Physician*. Military Medical Academy Publishing, St. Petersburg.

Poehl, A.V. (1903) Influence of catalysts on life and health of organism: spermine, cerebrine and adrenal-chloride. *Zhurn. med. khimii i organoterap*. **17**, 5–10; **27–29**, 1–30.

Poletaev, A.B. and Churilov, L.P. (2010) Immunophysiology, natural autoimmunity and human health. *Anosia* (*Immunity*). *Quart. Edit. Hellenic Soc. Immunol.* **6**(1), 11–18.

Rubner, M. (1908) Probleme des Wachstums und der Lebensdauer. *Wien. Mitt. Ges. Innere Med. und Kinderheilk.* **7**, 58–72.

Russian folk tales re-told by AN Tolstoy. Pravda Publishing, Moscow, 1985, p. 368.

Ružicka, V.T. (1922) Die protoplasmahysteresis und das verjüngungsproblem. *Deutsch. Medizin. Wochenschr*. **48**, 931–932.

Savchenko, I.G. (1891) On the question of immunity to anthrax. *Vrach* **5**, 132–134.

Schultz, E.A. (1914), cit. after: Anisimov V.N., Solov'yov M.V. *Evolution of Concepts in Gerontology*. Eskulap, St. Petersburg, 1999, p. 130

Semyonov, N.N. *The Chain Reactions*. Goskhimtechizdat, Leningrad, p. 555

Shereshevskiy, N.A. (1940) Senility and endocrine death. In: *Senility*. Ukr. Acad. of Sci. Publishing, Kiev, 1940, pp. 31–38.

Sinclair, D. and Guarente L. (2006) Unlocking the secrets of longevity genes. *Sci. Am.* **3**, 48–57.

Singh, R., Upadhyay, G. and Kumar, S. *et al.* (2003) Hypothyroidism alters the expression of Bcl-2 family genes to induce enhanced apoptosis in developing cerebellum. *J. Endocrinol.* **146**, 39–46.

Sirotinin, N.N. (1981) *Evolution of the Resistance and Reactivity of the Organism*. Moscow, Meditsina Publishing, 1981.

Skulachev, V.P. (2003) Aging and the programmed death phenomena. *Topics Curr. Genet.* **3**, 191–238.

Skulachev, V.P., Anisimov, V.N. and Antonenko, Y.N. *et al.* (2009) An attempt to prevent senescence: a mitochondrial approach. *Biochim. Biophys. Acta* **1787**, 437–461.

Slater S.D. (2010). The discovery of thyroid replacement therapy. In: *JLL Bulletin: Commentaries on the History of Treatment Evaluation*. Available from: http://www.jameslindlibrary.org/illu...nt-therapy.pdf (date of access: Feb. 15th 2013).

Smith, L.R., Bost, K.L. and Blalock, J.E. (1987) Generation of idiotypic and anti-idiotypic antibodies by immunization with peptides encoded by complementary RNA a possible molecular basis for the network theory. *J. Immunol.* **138**(1), 7–9.

Stroev, Yu.I., Churilov, L.P. and Vasil'ev, I.G. (2010) Quality of life and wellbeing of elderly people in St. Petersburg: problems and solutions. In: *Health, Wellbeing, Competence and Aging*, Hong Kong, Oct 23rd–24th, Chin. Univ. EPU Publishing, Hong Kong, 2010, p. 49.

Stroev, Y.I. and Churilov, L.P. (2011) Adolescent obesity with rose striae as a juvenile form of metabolic syndrome characteristic for marfanoid individuals and related to autoimmune thyroiditis. *J. Diabetes* **3**(1s), 39–40.

Stroev, Yu.I., Churilov, L.P. and Agapov, M.M. *et al.* (2011) The clinical pathophysiology of the early metabolic syndrome: pathogenetic roles of juvenile dyspituitarism, connective tissue dysplasiae and autoimmune thyroiditis. *Pathol. Physiol. Experim. Terap.* **3**, 3–15.

Tarkhanov, I.R. (1891) Lifespan of animals, plants and people.*Vestnik Evropy* **3**(6), 538–552.

Tjukin, V.P., Churilov, L.P. and Fionik, O.V. (2010) The Polymath of Silver Age: Alexander Bogdanov — Physician, Naturalist and Philosopher. I. Bogdanov as Theoretician. *Vestnik Sankt-Peterburg. University*, ser. 11. Meditsina. 1, 236–249.

Vernadskiy, V.I. (1975) *Thoughts of Naturalist: Space and Time in Alive and Non-alive Nature*. V. I.- Nauka Publishing, Moscow, p. 175

Voronoff, S. (1926) *Etude sur la Vieillesse et la Rajeunissement par la Greffe.* Doin Publishing, Paris.

Wang, J, Griggs, N.D. and Tung, K.S. *et al.* (1998) Dynamic regulation of gastric autoimmunity by thyroid hormone. *Int. Immunol.* **10**(2), 231–236.

Wang, R., Xu, C. and Zhao, W. *et al.* (2003) Calcium and polyamine regulated calcium-sensing receptors in cardiac tissues. *Eur. J. Biochem.* **270**, 2680–2688.

Weismann, A. (1882) *Űber die Dauer des Lebens*. Verlag von Gustav Fischer, Jena.

Williams, E.D. and Doniach, I. (1962) The post-mortem incidence of focal thyroiditis. *J. Pathol. Bacteriol.* **83**, 255–264.

Yegorov, Y.E. and Zelenin, A.V. (2011) Racing for cell immortality: telomeres, telomerase and the measure of health (a reflection on the award of the 2009 Demidov Prize in the field of Biology given to Alexey Matveevich Olovnikov). *Russ. J. Dev. Biol.* **42**, 53–56.

Zaichik, A.Sh. and Churilov, L.P. (2008) *General Pathophysiology with the Principles of Immunopathology*, 4th Ed. ElBi-SPb. Publishing, St. Petersburg.

Zaichik, A.Sh., Churilov, L.P. and Utekhin, V.J. (2008) Autoimmune regulation of genetically determined cell functions in health and disease. *Pathophysiology* **15**(3), 191–207.

Zalmanov, A.S. (1966) *The Secret Wisdom of Human Organism.* Nauka Publishing, Moscow-Leningrad.

Chapter 7

Promoting the Elderly Health in Hong Kong: Strategies and Actions

Wai Man Chan

Abstract

In the face of the aging population worldwide, the World Health Organization has advocated the life course approach to promoting active aging. In Hong Kong, the Elderly Commission is the advisory body on policy for elders and the Elderly Health Service (EHS) has been established in the Department of Health to enhance primary health care for the elderly. An evidence-based approach is adopted in both the clinical service for elders in the 18 Elderly Health Centres (EHC) and in the public health promotion programs delivered by the 18 Visiting Health Teams (VHT), with needs assessment, setting of priorities, and in-built evaluation. In the EHCs, a holistic, continuing and comprehensive approach with multidisciplinary input emphasizing health education and empowerment is shown to be effective for changing health related lifestyle behavioural risk factors and health outcome of elders. Similarly, the VHTs adopt a multi-modality, train-the-trainer, empowerment and skill enhancement approach with multi-disciplinary input, and are effective in making change among the various target groups like elders and elderly homes. Making use of diverse publicity and health promotional methods including production of books for sale, EHS will continue to evolve to meet the changing health needs of the elders in Hong Kong.

Keywords: Health of the Elderly; Primary Health Care; Lifestyle; Public Health Promotion.

7.1 Aging of the Population

Like many countries in the world, Hong Kong is facing aging of the population. This is the consequence of two major factors: high life expectancy, and low birth rate. For more than four decades, the life expectancy at birth has been steadily rising, reaching 80.3 years among males and 86.7 years among females in 2011. The crude birth rate, on the other hand, has dropped significantly from 35.0 per 1000 population in 1961 to 7.0 per 1000 population in 2003. The proportion of the population aged under 15 decreased from 40.8% in 1961 to 11.6% in 2011 while the proportion of persons aged 65 and above increased from 2.8% in 1961 to 13.3% in 2011. The aging trend will accelerate after 2011 as the post-war baby-boomers turn 65 (Census and Statistics Department, 2012).

7.2 The Aging Phenomenon

Many people view the aging trend as a threat. Myths abound: e.g. elders are invariably sick or demented; they are stubborn; they can't learn, can't change; they have no sex life; and most of them live in elderly homes. All these negative images are actually incorrect, as indicated by the real facts and statistics. Another often overlooked fact is that the coming cohort of elders will be quite different from the elders we see today. While the latter usually moved to Hong Kong in their young adulthood for work, the next generation of elders would mostly be born locally, with better education opportunities and better preventive health care in childhood.

Gro Harlem Brundtland, the previous Director-General of the World Health Organization, said this about aging in 1999 (Brundtland, 1999):

> "Population aging is first and foremost a success story for public health policies as well as social and economic development..."

As longevity is one of the universal pursuits of humankind, population aging should be seen as an achievement rather than a threat.

7.3 Policy on Elderly Care

In 1997, the Chief Executive of the Hong Kong Special Administrative Region (HKSAR) has made "Care for the Elderly" a Strategic Policy Objective of the Government of the HKSAR. The objective is to improve the quality of life of our elderly population and to provide them with a sense of security, a sense of belonging and a feeling of health and worthiness.

The Elderly Commission was established in the same year with its main task to provide advice to the Government of the HKSAR in the formulation of a comprehensive policy in caring for elders (HKSAR, 1997).

One of the first tasks taken up by the Elderly Commission was Healthy Aging, in line with the worldwide trend to view aging as a positive process full of opportunities and needs. Taking reference from the experience of other countries, as well as local circumstances, the Elderly Commission mapped out four strategic directions for the Healthy Aging Campaign launched in 2001, namely (Elderly Commission, 2001):

- promote personal responsibility;
- strengthen community action;
- create supportive environment; and
- improve image of aging.

7.4 Active Aging

In the document "Active Aging: A Policy Framework", released in 2002, the World Health Organization advocates "active aging", defined as the process of optimizing opportunities for health, participation and security in order to enhance quality of life as people age. The focus is not just physical, mental and social health and well-being, but also maintaining autonomy and independence. It recommends adopting the life course approach and taking actions throughout the lifespan to reduce the accumulation of health risks while enhancing protective factors among various determinants of health. This is especially relevant for non-communicable diseases (NCD) which are the major cause for disability and chronic health problem in old age (WHO, 2002).

In Hong Kong, the health of the present cohort of elderly is not so good. Among community dwelling elders aged 60 and above, 70% suffer from chronic illness, the most common being hypertension (62.5%), diabetes (21.7%), hypercholesterolemia (16.3%) and ischemic heart disease (14.5%) (Census and Statistics Department, 2009). In another population study, it was found that 9.3% of elders aged 70 and above suffer from different degrees of dementia (Ng and Chan, 2009). Unlike communicable diseases with a clearly defined causative agent, these diseases take a long time to develop and multiple factors are involved. As behaviour and lifestyle factors like smoking, physical activity and eating habits have vital roles to play, it is necessary to help prevent and control these diseases through interventions on lifestyle factors.

7.5 Health Promotion

Health promotion is defined as the process of enabling people to take control over and to improve their health for the prevention of diseases and the attainment of optimal health and well-being. In addition to imparting knowledge and skills, health promotion also includes measures to create a conducive environment for desirable behaviours and other favourable health determinants such as social support and healthy public policies. With the ultimate objective to reduce inequities in health, a risk-based approach is often adopted whereby health promotion efforts are targeted towards those at higher risks.

Health promotion interventions should be evidence-based. The planning process should include needs assessment to identify the priority areas, the resources available, the possible options and the relevant influencing factors before selecting the strategy for action. Evaluation should form part of the intervention program to ensure effectiveness. Outcome measures can include health outcomes (e.g. reduced morbidity), behaviour outcomes (e.g. decreased smoking), social outcomes (e.g. improved quality of life) and capability outcomes (e.g. enhanced knowledge and skills).

7.6 Elderly Health Service

The Elderly Health Service (EHS) was established in 1998 with the mission to enhance primary health care for the elderly, improve their self-care ability, encourage healthy living and strengthen carer support so as to minimize illness and disability. Health promotion is part and parcel of the services provided by the 18 Elderly Health Centres (EHC) and 18 Visiting Health Teams (VHT).

Adopting the family medicine approach, which emphasizes on holistic care, continuity, teamwork and multidisciplinary input, EHCs provide comprehensive primary care which incorporates all three levels of prevention: health risk assessment and health education (primary prevention), early detection of diseases (secondary prevention), and enhancement of self-care ability (tertiary prevention). The EHCs operate on a membership basis, with an annual enrolment fee of $110. Each enrolled elder undergoes a health assessment and subsequent re-enrolment annually is voluntary.

7.7 Health Assessment

The objective of the health assessment is to screen for risk factors as well as diseases. It comprises four components, namely, health interview, screening tests, physical examination, and laboratory investigations. The in-depth health interview is conducted by a trained nurse by way of a questionnaire, which obtains information on the sociodemographic characteristics, social factors (social support and financial situation), life-styles factors (smoking history, alcohol use, exercise and dietary habits), physical health (fall history and existing medical conditions) as well as activities of daily living of the client. Screening tests on balance, visual acuity, hearing, depression and cognitive function are conducted, so are the waist circumference, height and weight for calculating the BMI (body mass index). Based on the findings of the health interview, a physical examination is then carried out by a doctor. Baseline biochemical tests are arranged, with additional radiological and other investigations as may be indicated clinically.

7.8 Follow-Up Care

Elders with health risk or problems identified during health assessment are provided with targeted, intensive, face-to-face health education delivered by nurses. The health education emphasizes on practical tips and is delivered with a multimodality approach, including health talk and support group (using standardized education kits and materials produced with multidisciplinary input), and individual counseling by the same nurse, with telephone follow-ups as needed. Clients with needs, e.g. those with fall risk, depressive mood or functional impairment, will be assessed, managed and counseled by in-house allied health professionals (dietitian, physiotherapist, occupational therapist, clinical psychologist), while those requiring specialist care, e.g. cancer detected during health assessment, are referred accordingly.

7.9 Measuring Health Outcomes

To assess the effectiveness of the intensive health education efforts, the dataset containing records of 22,513 EHC members (8396 males and 14,117 females) who enrolled for the first time between 2001 and 2003 was analyzed. Members found to have lifestyle risk factors of smoking, obesity or having inadequate exercise, or health problems of fall, depressive mood or functional impairment at the first health assessment were tracked serially for any change in the prevalence of these risk factors/ health problem in their subsequent four health assessments till 2007.

Improvement in lifestyle risk factor or health problem was observed for all five types of elders during follow-up, which continued in subsequent health assessments. Among the 2229 current smokers at baseline, the number of quitters continued to increase (Fig. 7.1). Among the 7024 members found to have inadequate exercise at baseline, there was a continuous increase in the number of those having adequate exercise (Fig. 7.2). Among the 1228 members found to be obese at baseline, more and more became non-obese subsequently (Fig. 7.3). Among the 2289 members who had fallen more than once at baseline, significant improvement was observed during follow-up visits (Fig. 7.4). Among the 1961 members found to be depressed at baseline, significant improvement was observed during the follow-up (Fig. 7.5). Among the 1506 members with functional impairment at their first health assessment, many became impairment-free at subsequent visits (Fig. 7.6).

These findings show that a holistic, continuing and comprehensive approach with multidisciplinary input emphasizing health education and empowerment is effective for changing health related lifestyle behavioural risk factors and health outcome of elders, hence dispelling myths that elders cannot change or are unwilling to change. The observation of changes over a period of up to six years also demonstrates the cumulative effects of health education efforts.

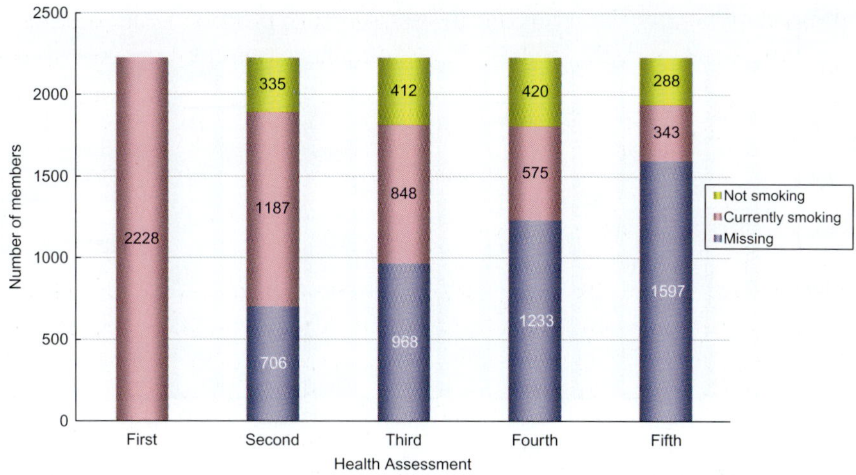

Figure 7.1. Change in smoking status of the smokers.

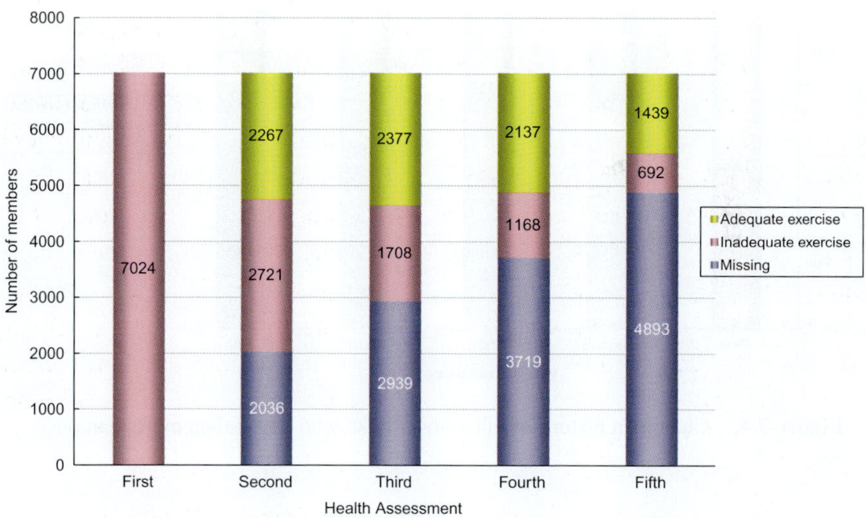

Figure 7.2. Change in exercise habit of those having inadequate exercise.

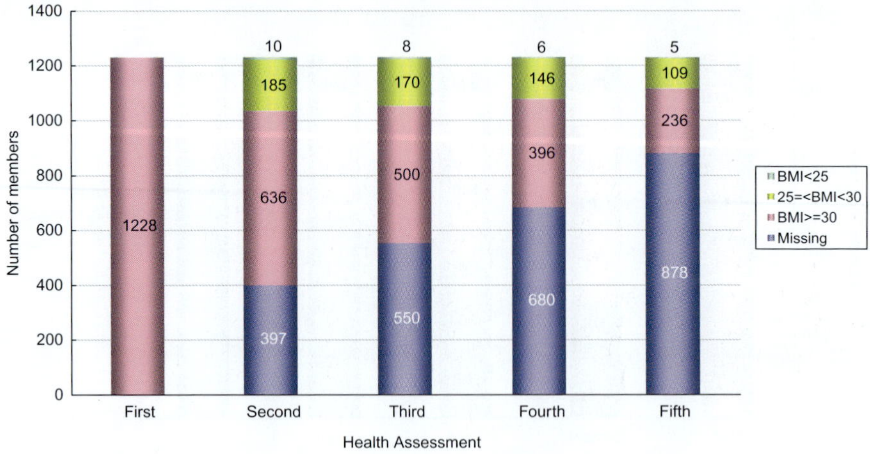

Figure 7.3. Change in BMI of the obese.

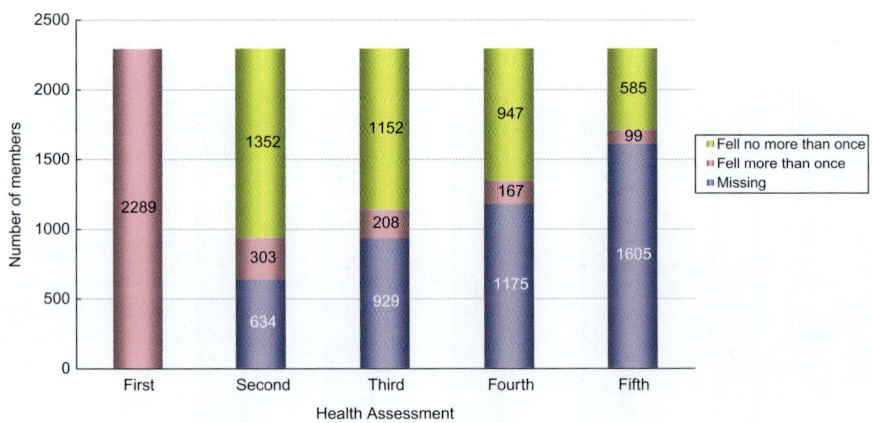

Figure 7.4. Change in history of fall among those who have fallen more than once.

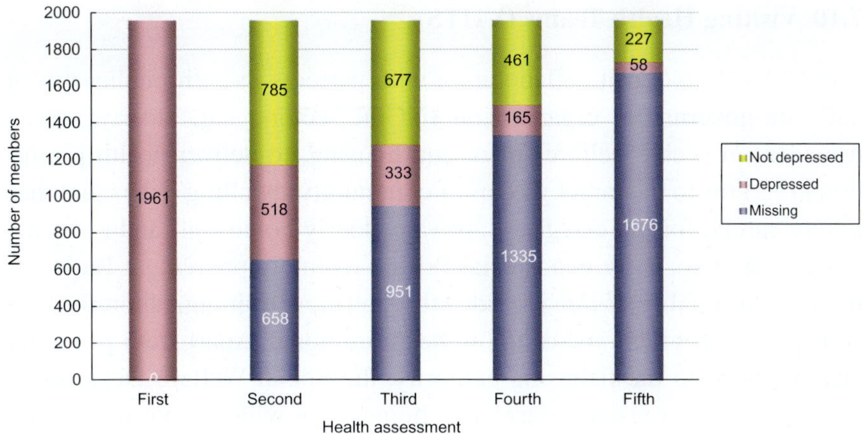

Figure 7.5. Change in depressive symptoms among the depressed.

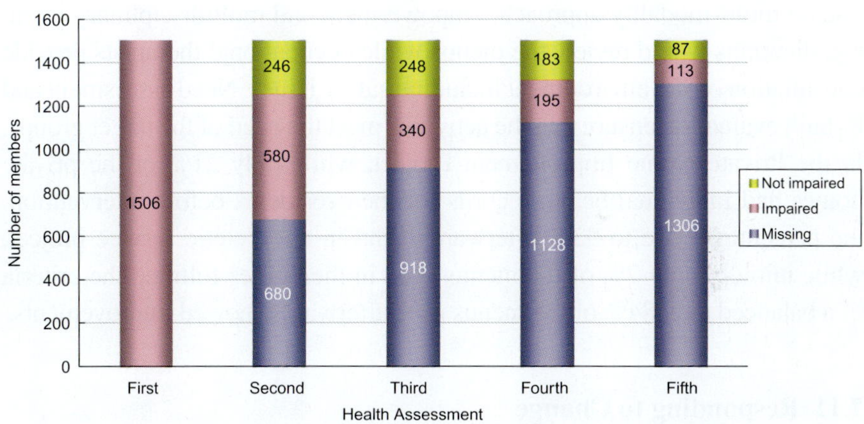

Figure 7.6. Change in functional status of those with impairment.

7.10 Visiting Health Teams (VHTS)

The 18 VHTs work in collaboration with partners in both public, private and non-government organization (NGO) sectors, e.g. elderly service providers in social welfare sector and housing, to deliver health promotion programs to the target groups of community-dwelling elders and their family carers, formal caregivers, private elderly home staff and residents. For the last two, there is a special Private Home Improvement Project to improve the quality of care provided through carer training, tailored advice and special programs focusing on the entire home. Apart from providing health advice to the licensing authority, the Social Welfare Department, VHTs pay regular visits to the elderly homes to provide on-site and tailored advice on various topics like nursing skills, exercise, and infection control. They also conduct annual assessment at all elderly homes to monitor progress and refine health education goals for the homes.

Similar to EHCs, the outreach health education programs of VHTs emphasise on multi-modality approach, empowerment and multidisciplinary input, e.g. dietitians would review the menus while occupational therapists provide consultation on the environment including safety issues. Need assessment and in-built evaluation ensure that the activities meet the need of the target groups. In the Private Home Improvement Project, while only 21% of the private homes had individual health records for their residents before intervention; the percentage rose to 93% afterwards. And in the dietetic service project, while initially only 7% of the menus used in the homes fulfilled the criteria of a balanced diet, 84% of the menus used afterwards showed improvements.

7.11 Responding to Change

Over the years, the VHT activities have evolved to meet changing needs and demands. With the SARS epidemic affecting many elders from elderly homes, EHS stepped up the health advice on infection control. SWD was advised to require all elderly homes to set up an infection control officer, and a set of guideline on prevention of communicable diseases was developed. On-site training, workshop and annual refresher course have now become on-going events, and a video on infection control practice has been produced and widely disseminated for ready reference.

Likewise, when there was much concern for the drug incidents in elderly homes, a guideline on drug management in elderly homes was developed after a need assessment survey. On-site advice, workshops and seminars were arranged, with on-going monitor to assess effectiveness.

7.12 Expert Advice and Resource Support

EHS actively supports the Elderly Commission's health-related deliberations. For the Healthy Aging Campaign, two special projects were developed: structured exercise for elders, and dietetic service for elderly homes. Apart from providing medical and health advisory input, EHS also provides resource support: two resource books on physical health and psychosocial health were produced, in addition to leaflets and videos on positive aging and structured exercises for both well and frail elders.

7.13 Elder Academy

More recently, Elderly Commission has launched the Elder Academy Scheme to promote Active Aging. This is a school-based elder learning program characterized by cross-sectoral collaboration and inter-generational harmony. It aims to promote continuous learning among elders, encourage them to widen their social networks, maintain physical and mental well-being and foster a sense of worthiness while acquiring knowledge. Each academy comprises a school collaborating with an elderly service provider, and health topic is mandatory in the curriculum (Labour and Welfare Bureau, 2012).

EHS provides input on the content of course materials, participates in the train-the-trainer program for potential instructors, and provides resource books for the instructors. All elder academies are also advised to make use of the books produced by EHS for reference in their classes on health topics.

7.14 Carer Training and Neighbourhood Active Aging Project

EHS supports the Carer Training and Neighbourhood Active Aging Project of the Elderly Commission. This project aims to train and make available a pool of "elder" sitters so as to give respite to informal elder carers in the community. It also promotes volunteer support to "hidden" elders in the neighbourhood. EHS provides input on the topics and the content of the training materials.

7.15 From Research to Program

Health promotion interventions should be evidence-based. In EHS, the four steps of need assessment, priority setting, implementation and evaluation are part and parcel of service mode. Operation research can be readily undertaken in the EHC platform, e.g. it is well known that aquatic exercise is beneficial for elders with osteoarthritis of the knees. However, it is unclear if the practice is acceptable to the more reserved elders in Hong Kong who usually do not know how to swim. A study was undertaken among EHC members, making use of public swimming pools. After demonstrating success in efficacy (reducing pain and improving performance), acceptability and feasibility, EHS now promotes the practice among NGOs and has produced a DVD to facilitate self-learning by elders with need.

7.16 Media Publicity

For public health education via media channels, EHS enjoys good relationship with partners and is regularly featured in a television program (TVB), a radio program (RTHK) and a newspaper for the elderly "The Voice". EHS operates a telephone hotline, a well-patronized webpage and a newsletter, and conducts press briefings from time to time, e.g. to promulgate the findings of a dementia prevalence study so as to arouse awareness for this disease.

7.17 Health Education Resource Materials

Over the years, EHS has produced a great number of health education resource materials like leaflets and VCD/DVDs, the latter two for sale at low cost. Health education kits originally designed for use by VHTs in the conducting of health education programs have also been adapted for other purposes, e.g. as fact sheets on EHS webpage and scripts for health columns in newspapers. To facilitate NGOs in conducting health education programs, many of them have been modified into DIY (do-it-yourself) kits and put on the webpage for free download (Elderly Health Service DIY, 2012).

EHS is increasingly recognized as the authority on elderly health information. The resource materials are popular with elders, family members, service providers, and also trainers. To provide more in-depth knowledge and understanding on various health topics, especially for the coming cohort of elders who are better educated with higher expectations for health information, EHS has started to produce books. These adopt the same approach of being holistic, comprehensive, with multidisciplinary input, and focus on prevention as well as quality of life. They help to widen the audience-ship of the EHS health education materials, reach new target groups, fill the market gap on certain health messages and promote public-private partnership. So far, nine books on six different topics have been produced and have proved to be very popular, with thousands of copies being sold (Elderly Health Service, 2012).

7.18 Future

For the future, EHS will continue to evolve. With its mission to provide quality primary health care services for promoting the health of our elderly population, EHS will strive to meet the need of the changing elders in Hong Kong, in accordance with its mission and values, which are:

- professionalism;
- client focus;
- whole-person, multidisciplinary team approach;
- continuous improvement;
- partnership in health; and
- proactive approach.

References

Census and Statistics Department. (2009) Socio-demographic Profile, Health Status and Self-care Capability of Older Persons, August 2009. http://www.statistics.gov.hk/publication/stat_report/social_data/B11302402009XXXXB0100.pdf

Census and Statistics Department. (2012) http://www.census 2011.gov.hk/pdf/main-report-volume-1.pdf

Department of Health. (2009) Dementia in Hong Kong, Public Health and Epidemiology Bulletin, Dec 2009. http://www.chp.gov.hk/files/pdf/bulletin_v18_n3_23122009.pdf

Elderly Health Service DIY. (2012) 自助式健康自學 / 教材套 [in Chinese] http://www.info.gov.hk/elderly/chinese/foreword-c.htm

Elderly Commission. (2011) Report on Healthy Aging, April 2001. http://www.elderly-commission.gov.hk/en/library/ROHA.HTM

Elderly Health Service. (2012) Book available at http://www.info.gov.hk/elderly/publications/cbook.htm

Labour and Welfare Bureau. (2012) http://www.elderacademy.org.hk/en/welcome/secretary.html

Speech by Dr. G.H. Brundtland, Director-General, World Health Organization, on World Health Day, 7 April 1999. http://www.who.int/director-general/speeches/1999/english/19990407_world_health_day.html

The 1997 Policy Address. (1997) the HKSAR Government, 8 Oct 1997.

World Health Organization. (2002) Active Aging, A Policy Framework, http://whqlibdoc.who.int/hq/2002/WHO_NMH_NPH_02.8.pdf

Chapter 8

Integrative Medicine and Anti-Aging in Japan

Kazuhiko Atsumi

Abstract

About 5000 years, the major traditional medicines were created: Chinese medicine, Ayurveda and Unani, in China, India and the Arab region, respectively.

In order to realize the medical dreams of personalized and preventive medicine, and also to solve problems such as economical and social educational matters, modern Western medicine is integrated with traditional medicine (TM) and complementary and alternative medicine (CAM) — collectively termed as integrative medicine. In this chapter, the key elements such as TM, CAM and their models and problems will be discussed.

Keywords: Integrative Medicine; Anti-Aging; Traditional Medicine; Chinese Medicine; Kampo; Ayurveda; CAM; Pulse Diagnosis; Meditation; Model of Integrative Medicine.

8.1 History of Medicine

About three million years ago, humans first appeared on the globe. Since then, humans have been suffering from health troubles due to hunger, cold, diseases and accidents. However, at that time, no science and no medicine existed, and patients had no way to cure themselves and could only to pray to God. In ancient days, religion took an important role in caring for patients. Some pioneers of medicine had tried food and natural herbs, etc. for healing. These experiences accumulated, resulting in traditional medicine in China, India and Arabs. These experiences and knowledge have been constructed and became Chinese medicine, ayurveda and unani medicine, respectively.

The information on these traditional medicines has been exchanged with each other and amalgamated, then delivered to the Europe. These transferred medicines had been constructed to the original initiative and European medicine was thus formed. Time passed and at the end of the 19th century, remarkable discoveries such as disinfection, blood transfusion and anesthesia were achieved and applied in surgery. These experiences and knowledge enhanced science and technologies of modern western medicine. In the 20th century, the wonderful technologies such as X-ray, ECG, blood chemical analysis and chemotherapy enabled the modernization of western medicine. In the 21st century, advanced technologies such as gene therapy, regenerative medicine and robotic surgery, etc., were developed and will be applied. Then, in the future, integrative medicine will be realized (Fig. 8.1).

8.2 Anti-Aging

Modern medical approaches have been done for anti-aging such as hormone replacement, enhancement of immunological powers, anti-free

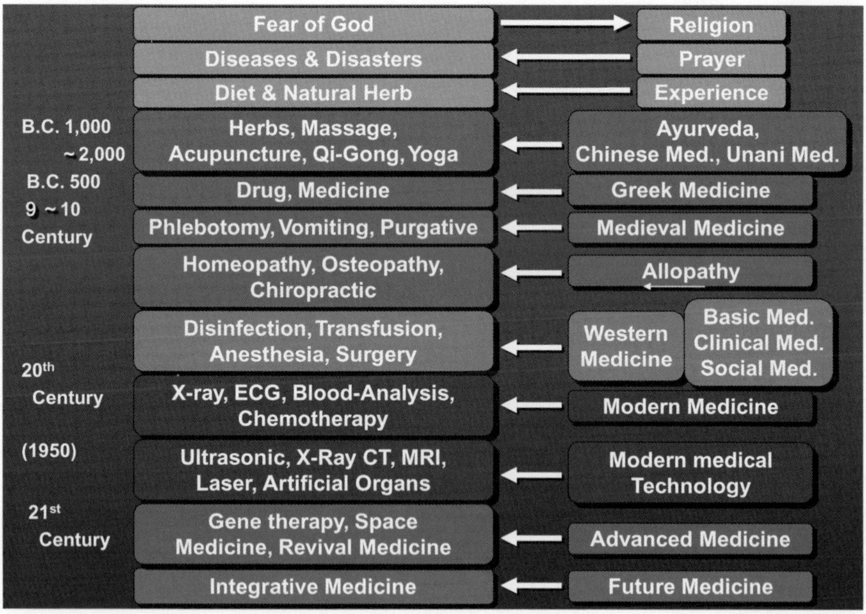

Figure 8.1. History of medicine.

radical therapy, organ transplantation, artificial organs, gene therapy, regenerative medicine, etc. However, an integrative medical approach on anti-aging will be using not only these modern approaches but also complementary and alternative medicine (CAM) and traditional medicine (TM) such as herbs, acupuncture, yoga, etc.

8.3 Integrative Medicine

The definition of integrative medicine is to integrate modern western medicine with CAM and TM. Modern western medicine (MWM) is based upon science and is considered as statistical medicine. On the other hand, CAM is based on experiences and is known as individual medicine. The two different health care systems will be integrated through evidence-based methods and tailored by gene-analysis, creating a the new system of integrated medicine (Fig. 8.2). Medicine is a nation's culture and CAM is different in each regions, depending on their foods, weather, social customs, etc., and also some new content will be added following as the development of technologies and societies. Therefore, at the present state, the contents of CAM in the specific regions are identified, however, the contents will be gradually changed. Table 8.1 shows the classification on CAM in Japan. As the traditional medicine, kampo is

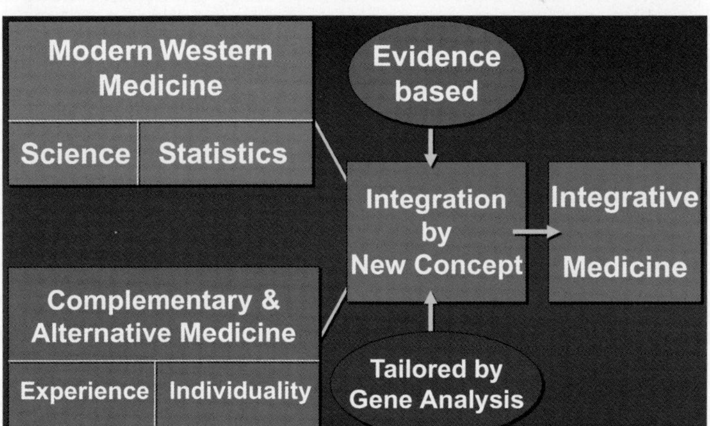

Figure 8.2. System of integrative medicine.

Table 8.1. Classification of CAM in Japan.

1) Traditional Medicine	4) Manual Therapy
• Kampo	• Shiatsu
• Chinese Medicine	• Massage
• Ayurveda	• Chiropractic
• Naturopathy	• Judo-Seifuku
• Acupuncture	• Reflexology
2) Life Style	**5) Mind-Body Therapy**
• Diet Therapy	• Psycho-Therapy
• Fasting Therapy	• Hypnosis
• Diet Supplement	• Bio-feedback Therapy
• Exercise	• Relaxation
3) Herb	• Meditation
• Kampo Herb	• Music Therapy
• Various Herbs	• Humor Therapy

unique in Japan. Fasting therapy is used. In manual therapy, shiatsu and judo-seifuku are unique in Japan.

8.4 Traditional Medicine (TM)

Table 8.2 shows the major traditional medicines in the world. Under Japan, kampo, acupuncture, shiatsu, judo-seifuku, hot spring and meditation are listed. Under China, Chinese medicine, Tibet medicine, acupuncture, Chinese herb, qigong, etc., are listed. In India, Ayurveda and yoga are listed. In Arab, unani medicine is listed. In Europe and the US, acupuncture, herb, chiropractic, naturopathy and homeopathy are listed.

8.4.1 *Chinese medicine*

As the most typical and popular traditional medicine, traditional Chinese medicine (TCM) is introduced. The principle of Chinese medicine has been based on the views "How to understand universe" and "How to recognize the human body as a small universe".

The existence of human is harmonized in nature and universe. Chinese medicine started about 5000 years ago; at that time knowledge of science and medicine has never existed. Therefore, the name of organs in the human

Table 8.2. The major traditional medicines in the world.

Country & Region	Contents of Traditional Medicine
Japan	Kampo, Acupuncture & Moxibustion, Shiatsu, Judo- Seifuku, Hot Spring, Healthy Food
China, Taiwan	Chinese Medicine, Acupuncture & Moxibustion, Tibet Medicine, Mongol Medicine, Taichi, Qigon
India	Ayurveda Unani Medicine, Yoga
Arab	Unani Medicine
Europe	Aropathy, Homeopathy, Acupuncture, Hot Spring Therapy, Phytotherapy, Aromatherapy
Africa	Herb Etc.
USA	Native American Medicine, Chiropractics, Naturopathy, Reflexology

Table 8.3. Comparison of modern Western medicine vs. Chinese medicine.

	Modern Western Medicine	Chinese Medicine
Base & Mode	Science based, Statistical	Experience-based, Individual
Unit	Cell, Molecule	Qi, Five Elements
Organ	Modern Anatomy	Chinese Philosophy
Diagnosis & Therapy	Same Therapy with Same Diagnosis	Different Therapy with Same Diagnosis
Drug vs. Herb	Effect of Identified Chemical Substances	Integrative Effect, not Identified Scientifically
Standardization	Easy	Difficult

body is not identified as the same organs in the present modern western medicine. The functions of the internal organs are also defined differently in Chinese medicine compared to modern western medicine. The essential factors of philosophy of Chinese medicine consists of "*qi*" (bio energy), "*yin* and *yang*" and five "*gogyo*" (the five actions or elements), etc. (Table 8.3).

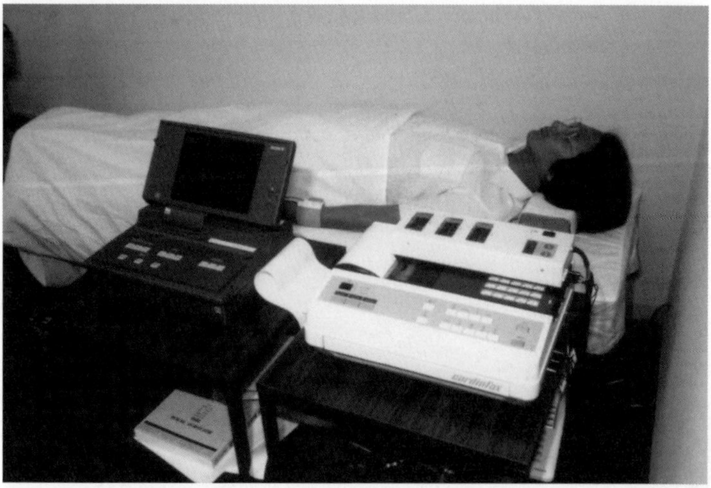

Figure 8.3. The pulse diagnosis device by Sony company.

Western medical doctors can make cardiovascular diagnosis from radial pulse information, such as arteriosclerosis and arrhythmia; however, Chinese medical doctors can make holistic diagnosis on whole body conditions by pulse diagnosis.

We constructed a pulse diagnostic device with the software of Chinese medicine utilizing audio sensors by Sony company.

Three pulse sensors — sensitive microphones — were used. These sensors were set on the patient's radial artery and the sounds were recorded by the reorder. (Figs. 8.3 and 8.4).

Figure 8.5 shows the three amplitude patterns detected from the sensors. From upper portion, the proximal, central and distal patterns were indicated.

Figure 8.6 shows one of the characteristics of the blood flow recorded by pulse diagnosis sensors.

Figure 8.7 shows the one of case of pulse change of a patient before and after dialysis treatment.

Applying the device, a lot of holistic information on human body, for the clients and patients wes obtained. It's considered that the device will be useful to evaluate the efficacy in anti-aging and CAM research.

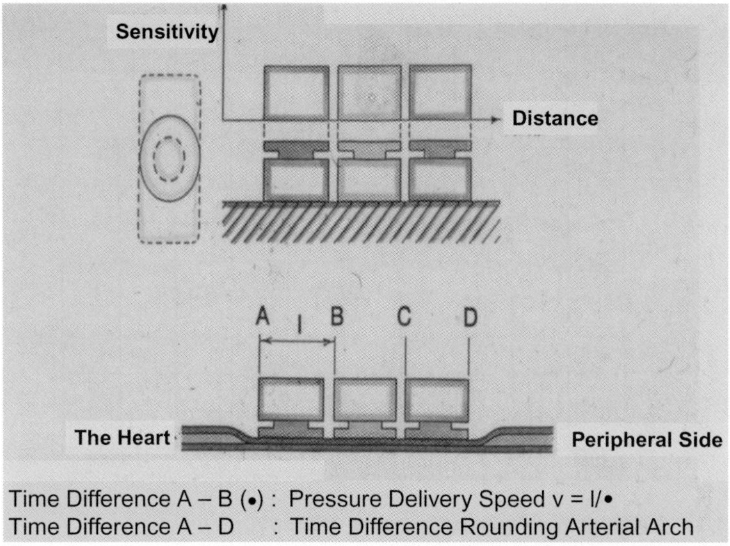

Figure 8.4. Characteristics of three pulse sensor.

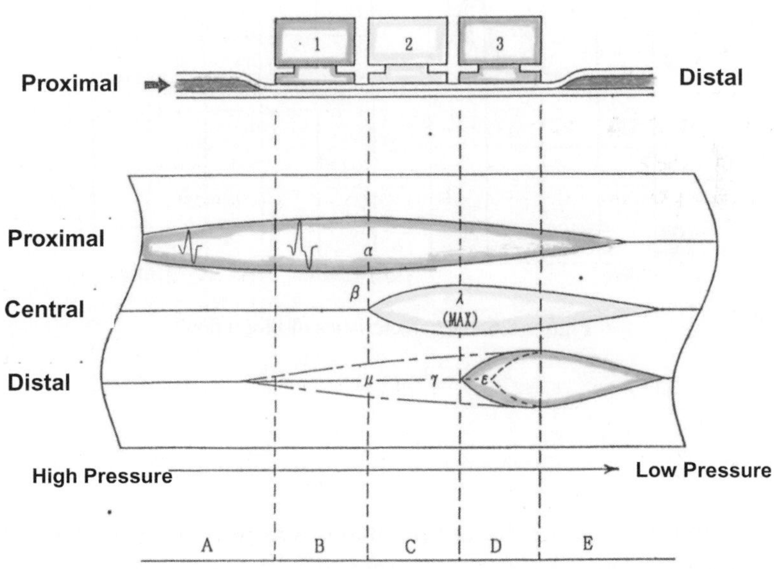

Figure 8.5. Three amplitude patterns from three sensors.

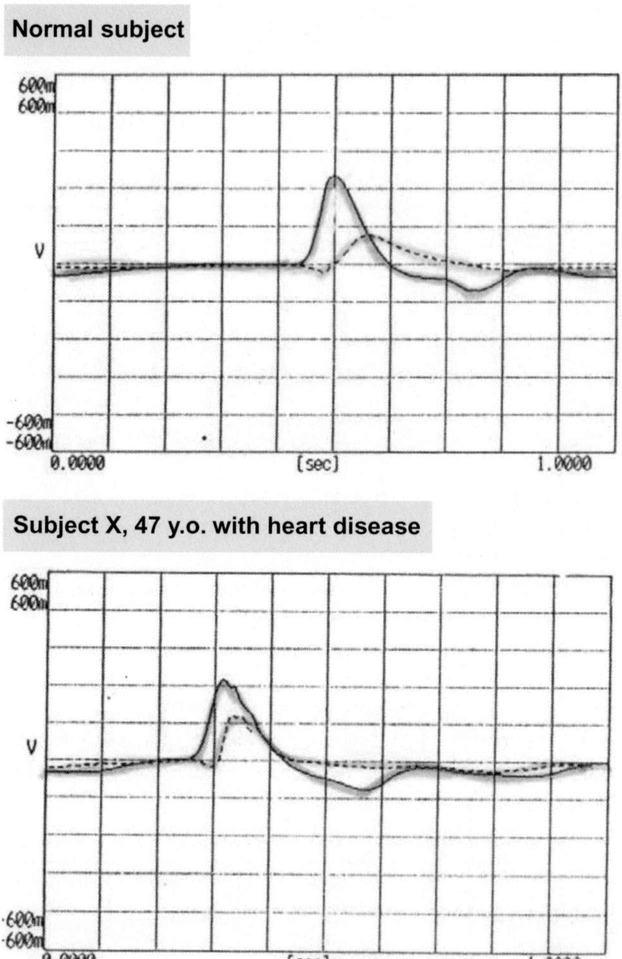

Figure 8.6. Characteristics of blood flow.

8.4.2 *Kampo*

About 1000 years ago, Chinese medicine was introduced to Japan from China by Buddhists. It was amalgamated with Japanese folk medicine, creating kampo, which was considered to have developed to a different system from Chinese medicine.

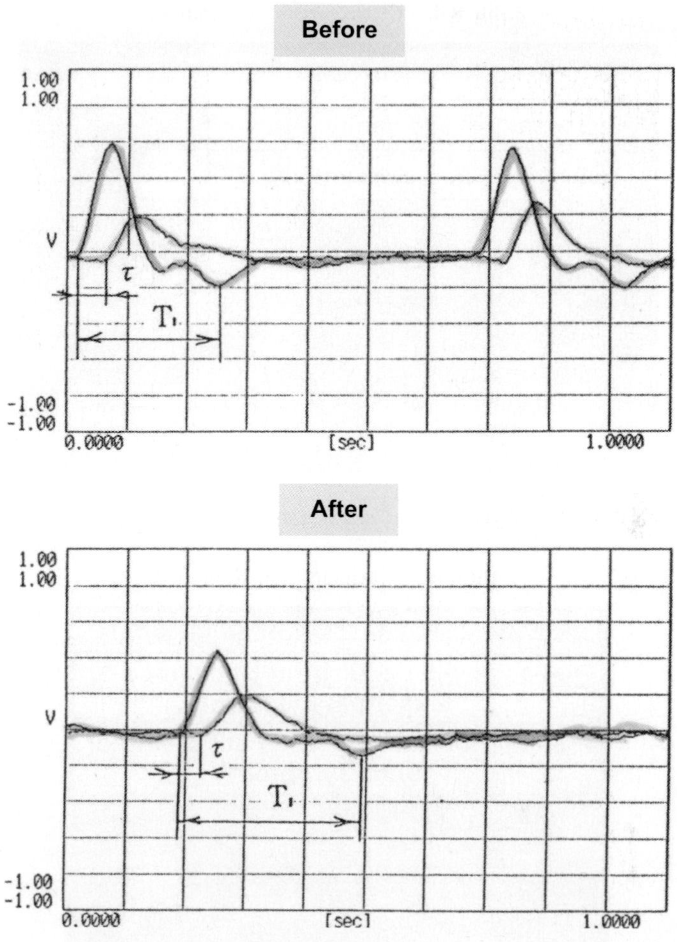

Figure 8.7. The pulse changes before and after dialysis treatment.

At the present state, about 200 species of kampo herbs approved by the Japanese Government. The formulas are highly evaluated in quality control in production processes worldwide.

From a questionnaire survey in 2000, 70% of Japanese doctors used kampo, 29% of patient's required and 22% of kampo herbs are used for lifestyle disorders.

The concept of the characteristics of kampo is shown in Table 8.4.

Qi, *sho*, five organs, *keiraku*, and *tsubo* are the same concepts with those of Chinese Medicine. The principles of kampo are shown in the

Table 8.4. Characteristics of Kampo.

Qi（気）、Keiketsu（血）、Sui（水）
Fullness（実）& Vanity（虚）
Positivity（陽）& Negativity（陰）
Sho（証）（Multiple Diagnosis）
Five Organs（五臓）
Liver（肝）、Heart（心）、Spleen（脾）、
Lung（肺）、Kidney（腎）、 Keiraku（経絡、Rout of Chi）& Keiketsu（経穴、Acupuncture points）

Table 8.5. Principles of Kampo.

Individual (Patient) Oriented Medicine
Diseases will occur from Unbalance of Essential Elements
Treatment will be decided according of Sho (Symptom)
Focusing on Preventive Care & Health Promotion rather than Therapeutics
Kampo Herb, Acupuncture, Herbal Diet, Exercise, Massage are Utilized as Therapeutic Tools

Table 8.5. It was originally the same as Chinese medicine, however, the diagnosis methods and the kampo herb species are different.

Figure 8.8 shows a difference between Chinese medicine and kampo. In Chinese medicine, from diagnosis to therapy, three complicated processes are necessary: analysis of pathological data, decision of therapy method, and consideration of therapy contents. However, in kampo, the process is simple: only the patient's constitution has to be identified to decide "sho" and therapy is automatically decided according to "sho".

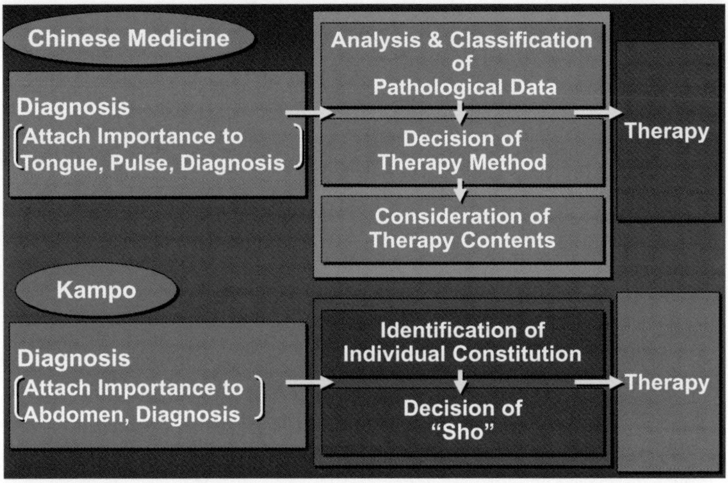

Figure 8.8. Differences between Chinese medicine and Kampo.

8.4.3 *Ayurveda*

Ayurveda is the Indian traditional medicine (Fig. 8.9).

In ayurveda, the three "*dosha*" — verta, pitta and kava — are the important factors with the five elements and related with the constitutions of individuals.

The relationship between dosha and disease and health are shown in Table 8.6. Patient health is promoted according to the grade of balance in the three doshas; in reverse, disease is worsened. Various kinds of the unique therapies can be used in ayurveda. Figure 8.10 shows "*sirodhara*", warmed oil down on the center of the forehead. Recently, Dr. Uebaba in Toyama University constructed a healing robot on sirodhara which control of oil volume and dropping speed automatically by computer.

8.5 Complementary and Alternative Medicine (CAM)

8.5.1 *Yoga*

Yoga is a well-known therapy to keep the body healthy using herbs, meditation and exercise, developed 4000 years ago in India (Fig. 8.11) Now, yoga is popular not only in young people but also in aged people

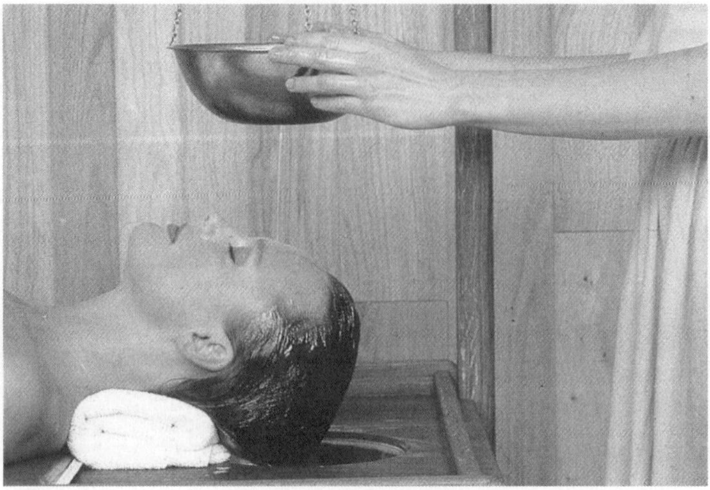

Figure 8.9. Ayurveda.

Table 8.6. Relationship between dosha, disease and health.

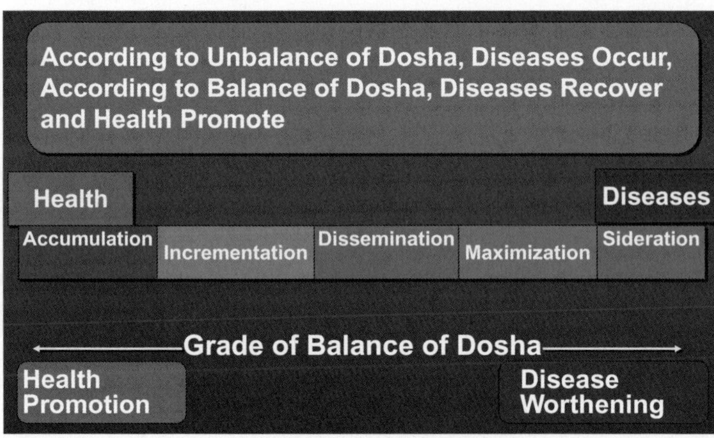

for anti-aging in Japan. Yoga is combined with psychosomatic therapy to relax patients physically and mentally, and their results have been reported in the medical conferences in Japan.

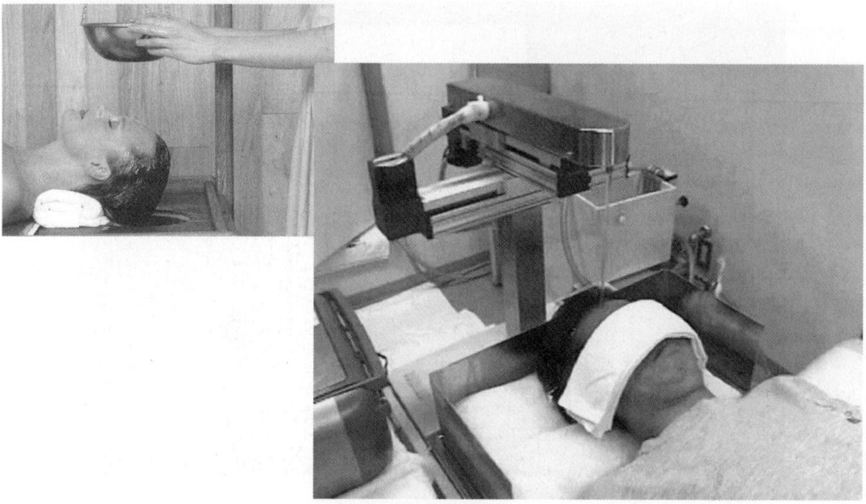

Figure 8.10. A healing robot on sirodhara.

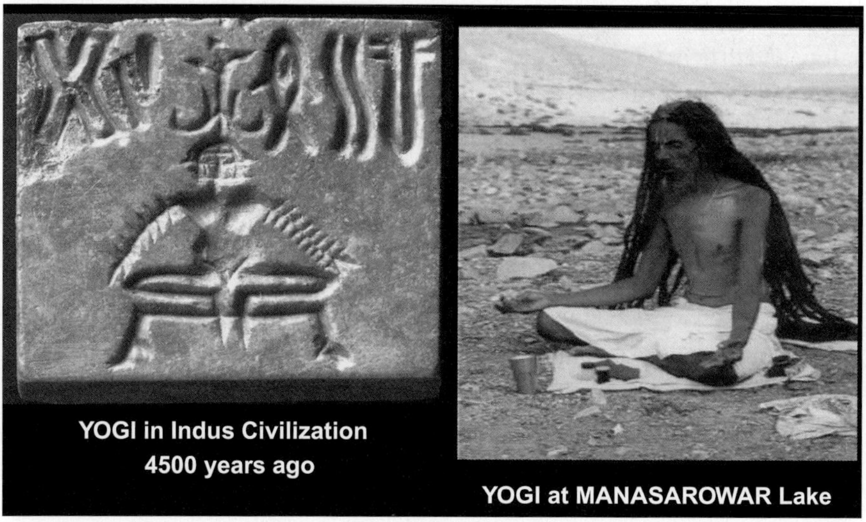
YOGI in Indus Civilization
4500 years ago
YOGI at MANASAROWAR Lake

Figure 8.11. Yoga.

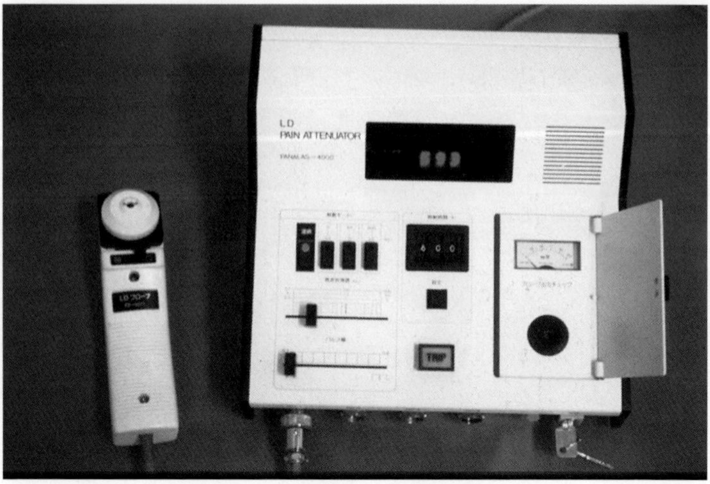

Figure 8.12. The diode laser for acupuncture.

8.5.2 *Acupuncture*

Acupuncture therapy has been widely used in Asian countries and the safety and efficacy have been approved by many reports. The World Health Organization (WHO) has reported guides on the effective applications of acupuncture for patients. Recently, semi-diode lasers with low power are used for acupuncture (shown in Fig. 8.12).

The medical results of laser acupuncture are considered as same as with conventional needle acupuncture. The application fields are wide in wound healing, pain relief, etc.

The effective mechanism has been studied in molecular level utilizing genome analysis in Japan. One of the cases of pain treatment for a patient of rheumatic arthritis by laser acupuncture is shown in Fig. 8.13.

8.5.3 *Qigong*

Qigong can use to keep healthy and to discover body ability by adjusting his/her own conditions. Qigong has been used in the aged people to strengthen physically and mentally, not only in China but also in Japan (Fig. 8.14).

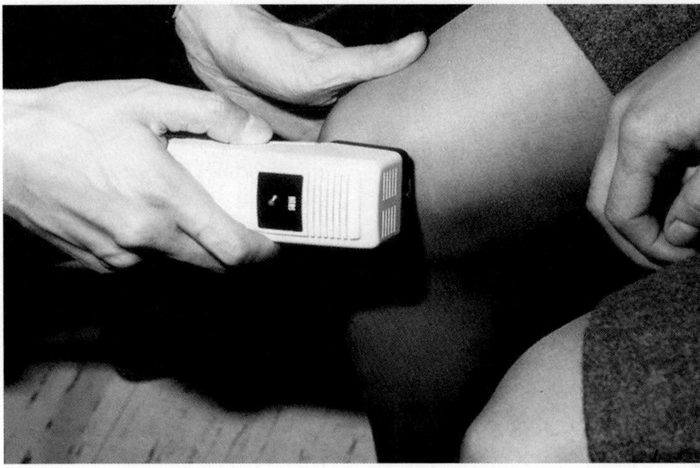

Figure 8.13. Treatment by laser acupuncture.

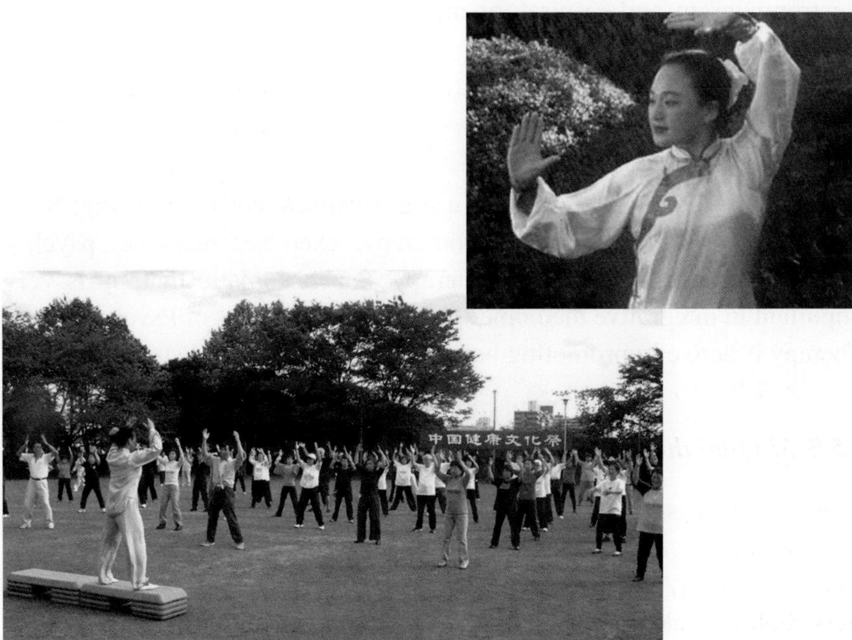

Figure 8.14. Qigong.

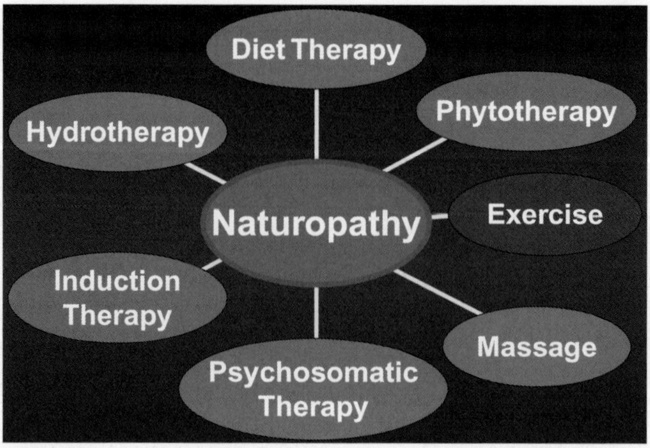

Figure 8.15. The various methods in naturopathy.

The effective mechanism was analyzed utilizing electroencephalogram, electromyogram and respiratory measurements in Tokyo Technological College.

8.5.4 *Naturopathy*

Naturopathy includes the various useful methods as shown in Fig. 8.15: hydrotherapy, diet therapy, phytotherapy, exercise, massage, psychosomatic therapy, and induction therapy. Psychosomatic therapy is very important in integrative medicine. The Japanese Society of Psychosomatic Therapy is active in promoting basic research and clinical study.

8.5.5 *Manual therapy*

Table 8.7 shows the comparison among the various manual therapies in naturopathy: *anma*, massage, *judo-seifuku*, chiropractic, *seitai*, *suikon*, reflexology, aromatherapy, etc. Wide techniques that are rub, chafe, smooth, lad, stroke vibrate, and the other methods have been used in message, *seitai*, *suikon*, reflexology and aromatherapy (Fig. 8.16, Table 8.7).

The applications' areas are wide in soft tissue, skeleton, joints and whole body.

Table 8.7. Comparison of the various manual therapies.

	Therapy	Amma	Massage	Judo Seifuku	Chiro-practics	Seitai	Suikon	Reflexology	Aroma-therapy
Therapeutic Method	Rub.	○	○		○	○	○	○	○
	Chafe		○			○	○	○	○
	Smooth		○			○	○	○	○
	Pad	○	○		○	○	○	○	○
	Stroke		○			○	○	○	○
	Vibrate		○			○	○	○	○
	Others			Treatment on Dislocation & Fracture		Reform on Skelton	〃	〃	Electric
Therapeutic Areas		Soft Tissue	Soft Tissue		Soft Tissue	Skelton & Joint	Skelton Joint, Soft Tissue	Low Extremities	Whole Body, Soft Tissue

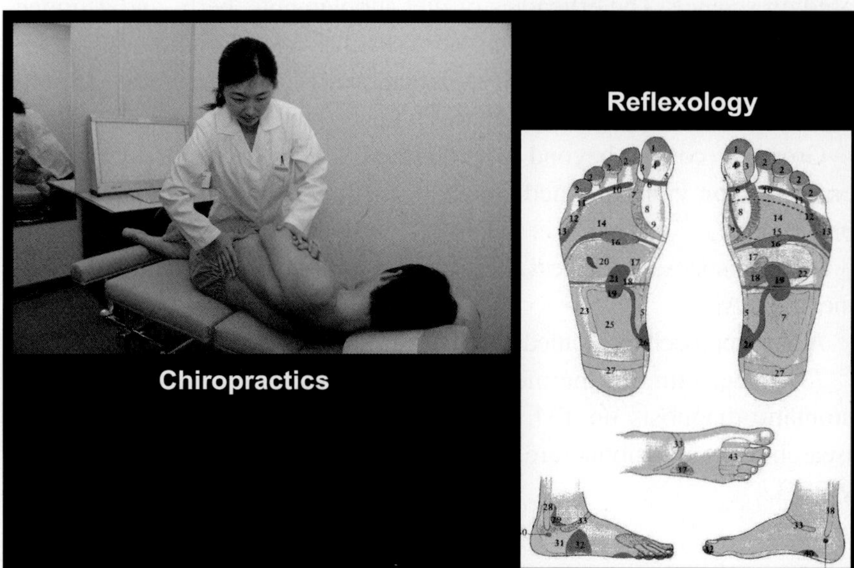

Figure 8.16. Manual therapy.

8.5.6 *Hot spring therapy*

In Japan, many volcanoes are present with some still active, therefore, many kinds of hot springs can be seen in the seaside and mountains in Japan. From ancient times, Japanese people have enjoyed hot springs, staying for a couple days with their families (Fig. 8.17).

It is considered that Japanese long life depends on the beneficial effects of hot springs.

Figure 8.18 shows the efficacy of hot springs for anti-aging. The physical, thermal and chemical effects, with exercise and natural environment, have contributed to bring integrative effects — physical and mental — and as a result, healthy and anti-aging effects are promoted

8.6 Scientific Approach to CAM/TM

The scientific approach to CAM/TM is divided into the three groups:

Group 1 can be clarified by traditional EBM methodologies which is based on science. The efficacies of diet supplements, herbs and acupuncture are included in the group.

Group 2 can be clarified by new evaluation method and analysis. The efficacy of music therapy, *qigong* and touch therapy are included in the group.

Group 3 covers beyond conventional scientific methodology. The verification on vibration medicine and spiritual healing are considered to be included.

It is indispensably necessary to make a bridge between modern medicine and CAM.

A new approach by biomedical engineering on CAM is shown in Fig. 8.19.

Tsubo detecting by thermograph with the hot spots by a wave in EEG, automatic diagnosis on TM, evidence of effect of meditation by EEG, research on laser acupuncture, pulse diagnosis device, and effect of *qigong* by EEG.

8.7 The Model of Integrative Anti-Aging Clinic

In order to promote anti-aging in integrative medicine, various kinds of models will be designed: clinic, hospital,l and regional planning.

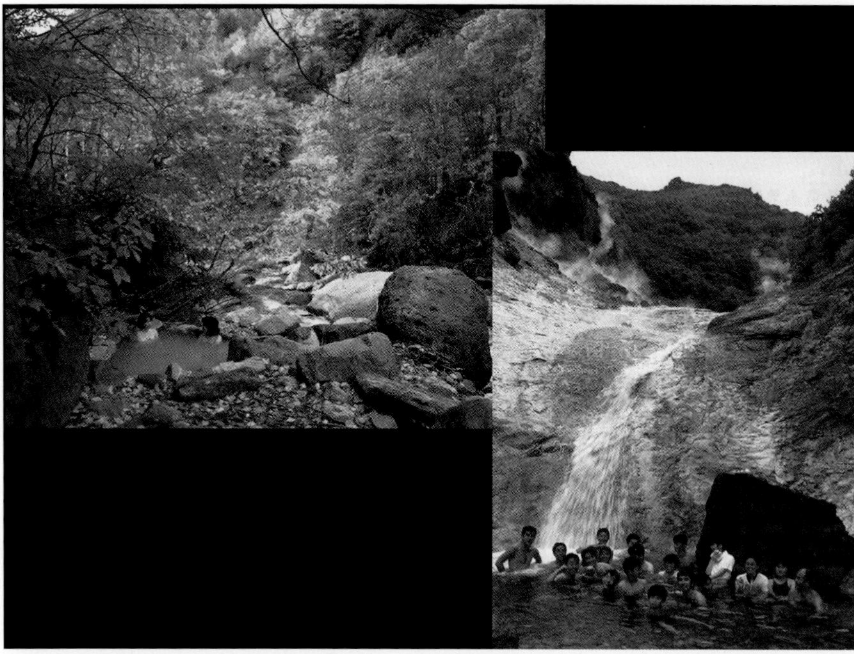

Figure 8.17. The Japanese enjoy hot springs during every season.

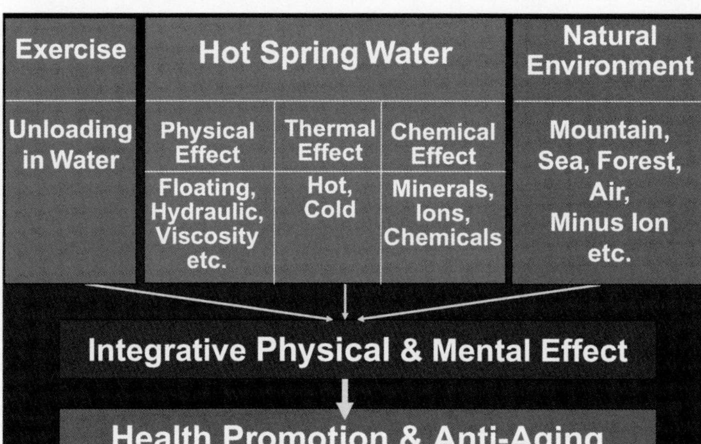

Figure 8.18. Efficacy of hot springs for anti-aging.

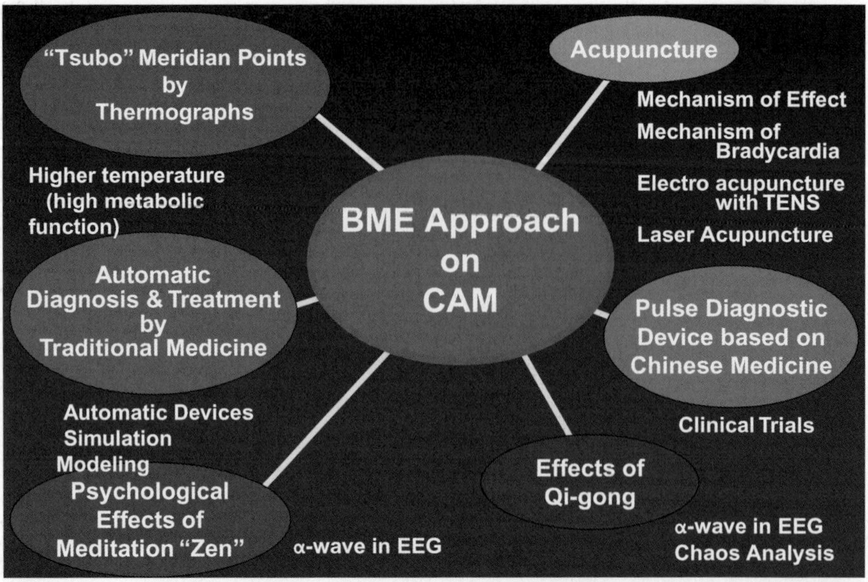

Figure 8.19. BME approach on CAM in Japan.

Figure 8.20 shows one of the models on an integrative anti-aging clinic.

The clinic is connected with the modern medical center, central institute for aging and computer center for database and various kinds of CAM and TM.

The physical and bio functional data are measured and also DNA and biomarkers are analyzed on the clients.

8.8 Regional Model for Integrative Medical Center

The larger-scale type, regional model is designed in Okinawa Island.

In the upper side of the Fig. 8.21, the academic medical facilities and institute are connected with the integrative medical center.

On the right side, CAM and traditional medical facilities such as kampo, ayurveda, Tibet medicine, homeopathy, naturopathy, acupuncture, massage, yoga, chiropractic, thalassotherapy, animal therapy and herbs, etc., are situated.

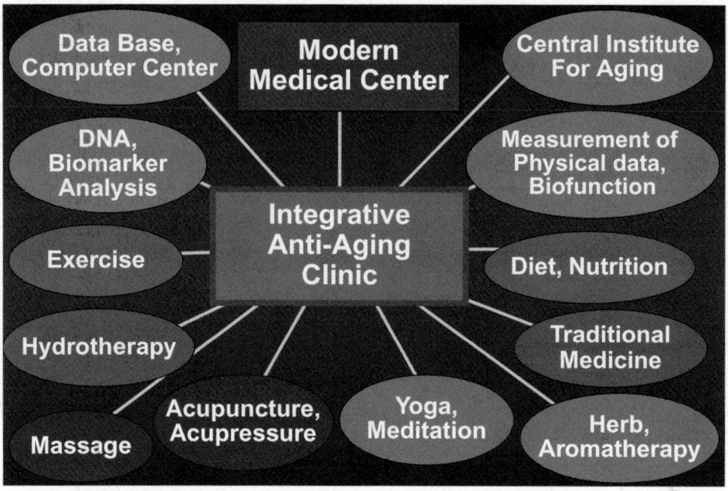

Figure 8.20. Network of integrative anti-aging clinic.

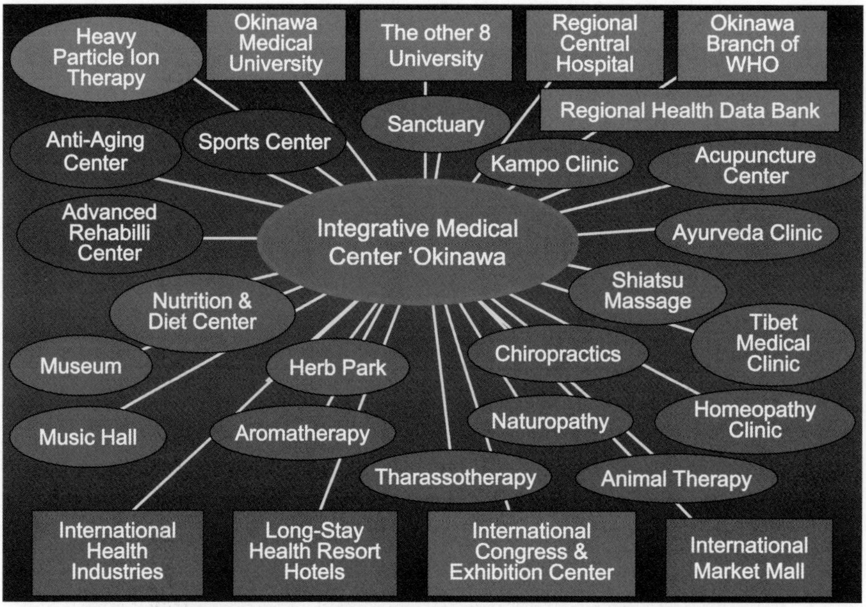

Figure 8.21. Concept of consortium on integrative medicine for anti-aging okinawa.

On the left side, the anti-aging center, rehabilitation center, sports center are situated. Also, the museum and music hall are connected and used as health resources.

At the bottom, health industries, long-stay resort hotels, international conference center and exhibition and market place are situated.

These facilities are connected with a network utilizing computers.

8.9 Future Medicine

Before my conclusion, I would like to introduce Hiroo Imura's paper, which compared medicine and health care in the 20th and the 21st centuries (Table 8.8).

In the 20th century, the method of science is expressed as reductionism; on the other hand, in 21st, it is expressed as integration.

In the 20th century, the key word was gene; however, in the 21st, it will be network.

In the 20th century, the mind and body ware considered to be separated; however, in the 21st, they will be integrated.

In the 20th century, the health care system has been developed as doctor-oriented and therapeutics-oriented; however, in the 21st, it will be oriented on team care and prevention, and integrative medicine will

Table 8.8. Comparison of medicine and healthcare in the 20th and 21st century.

	20th Century	21st Century
Method	Reductionism	Integration
Key Word	Gene	Network
Mind & Body	Separation	Integration
Medicine	Specialization	Generalization
Health Care	Doctor-Oriented Therapeutics	Team Care Prevention
	Modern Western Medicine	Integrative Medicine

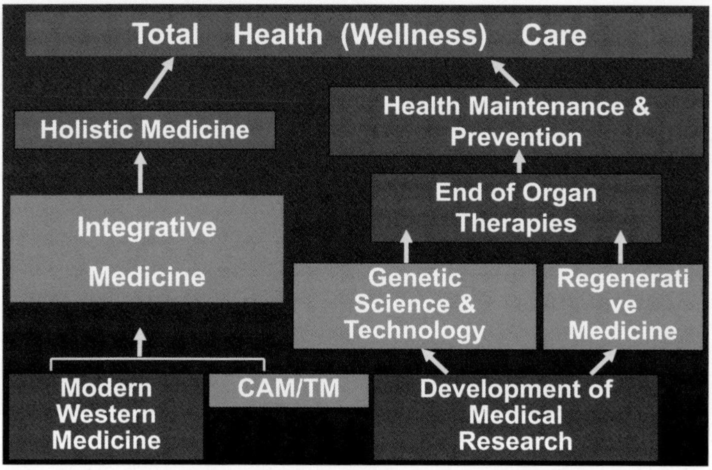

Figure 8.22. Towards future total health care.

become mainstream. Now I would like to mention future total health care, as shown in Fig. 8.22. In basic studies, the two major innovative development of genetic science and regenerative medicine will bring the end of therapies and through promotion, total health care will be realized. In the other hand, in clinical field, integrative medicine will be achieved and finally total health care will be realized.

8.10 Summary

The goal and objectives of integrative medicine are as follows:

(1) Anti-aging is one of the model of integrative medicine.
(2) Individual medicine will be achieved by integration of modern western medicine and CAM and traditional medicine, namely, by the approach of integrative medicine.
(3) Integrative medicine will become new ideal medicine and will create new techniques, new products and new industries.
(4) The innovative impact of integrative medicine will be strong and the human society will be changed evolutionally.

Chapter 9

Medical Resonance Therapy Music®

Dr. Ernest HM, Ma

Abstract

Medical Resonance Therapy Music® originated from Peter Hubner in Germany using the theory of resonance for applications in clinical settings by his multidisciplinary team of professionals. The sonic (20–2000 Hz) and subsonic frequency (0.034–5 Hz) of resonance music is best delivered through headphones with ear muffs in an undisturbed environment 20 minutes or more twice a day. Therapeutic music synchronizes with cellular physiological rhythm, restores neuro-hormonal balance and rekindles the body ability of auto-healing. It helps in restoring different physiological functions, including the nervous, circulatory, digestive and endocrine systems that have their own rhythms. With the appropriate frequency of music, users enter a state of relaxation that guides the body to adjust its pace to deal with stress, insomnia, anxiety, migraine headache, hypertension, hormonal and immune disorders and other clinical problems. The best known examples were serving victims of the Chernobyl nuclear plant incident and children with hypertension. In Germany nowadays, patients can buy Medical Resonance Therapy Music® CDs from pharmacies based on physician prescriptions for 18 types of common medical symptoms and problems, supported by over five years of positive clinical and scientific evidence.

Medical Resonance Therapy Music® should not be overlooked as its new developments have already expanded to Chinese Medicine like “acu-music” (music of different Meridians), Chiropractic practice (music for Spine health), Ayurvedic Medicine (music of Chakras energy centres), mindfulness based meditation (music of meditation) and education (whole brain nurture, creativity and intelligence). The strength of Western Medicine lies in cure of infectious diseases, surgeries and emergency life-saving. Chinese Medicine is strong in managing sub-health before diseases emerge. Natural Medicine goes back to basics of nature and adopts our self-healing power to promote health. However, Medical Resonance Therapy Music® should be considered as a complementary therapy of health problems, but not replacing evidence-based Western Medicines.

Keywords: Music Therapy; Resonance Music; Medicine; Acupuncture; Meridian.

Medical Resonance Therapy Music® originated from Peter Hubner in Germany using the theory of resonance for applications in clinical settings by his multidisciplinary team of professionals including musicians, acoustic scientists and clinicians. The sonic (20–2000 Hz) and subsonic frequency (2–15 Hz; as low as 0.034 Hz) of resonance music is best delivered through headphones with ear muffs, in an undisturbed environment 20 minutes or more twice a day. The therapeutic music synchronizes with cellular physiological rhythm, restores neuro-hormonal balance and rekindles the body ability of auto-healing (Chui, 2003).

Peter Hubner applied Medical Resonance Therapy Music® to improve physical problems by restoring different physiological functions, including the nervous, circulatory, digestive and endocrine systems that have their own rhythms. With the appropriate frequency of music, users enter a state of relaxation to guide the body to adjust its pace to deal with stress, insomnia, anxiety, migraine headache, hypertension, hormonal and immune disorders, and other clinical problems. The music is best known in serving victims of the Chernobyl nuclear plant radiation leak accident. In another study, children who suffered from hypertension improved after use of the music (Sidorenko, 2000a, b and c). In Germany nowadays, patients can buy Medical Resonance Therapy Music® CDs from pharmacies based on physician prescriptions of 18 types of common medical symptoms and problems. These scientific evidence would be illustrated (Lee, 2000).

The 18 common types of Western Medicine based Medical Resonance Therapy Music® CDs are listed below. RRR stands for relaxation, recreation and rejuvenation with efficacy supported by over five years of positive clinical evidence and scientific research. Indications for music preparation 18 RRR CDs (Peter Hubner, Germany) include:

- Headache/Migraine (RRR 133)
- Harmony (RRR 102), General Stress Symptoms (RRR932), Relaxation (RRR931)
- Sleep Disorders (RRR 106)

- Cardiac and Circulatory Disorders (RRR940)
- Pains/Post-Operative Pains (RRR 943)
- Neurodermatitis/Psoriasis (RRR933)
- Disorders of the Hormone and Immune System (RRR103)
- Neurophysiological and Sensory Disorders (RRR941), Concentration/Memory (RRR128), Creativity (RRR935)
- Mental Distress/Fear (RRR951), Courage to Face Life (RRR921), Vital Energy (RRR)
- Gynecological Disorders (RRR105), Pregnancy and Birth (RRR934), Mother and Child (RRR942)

The Medical Resonance Therapy Music® (MRT-Music) frequency ranges from> 20 Hz down to 0.034 Hz (simulating brainwaves) are constructed through 6-level digital technology with 256 soundtracks. This is in contrast to 2-level digital and 25 soundtracks in usual music CDs. Replicating MRT-Music with mp3 recording results in loss of the special effects and thus not recommended.

Clinical research findings in some common conditions are illustrated as follows (www.medicalresonancetherapymusic.com):

(1) Headaches (after ten days of 30–40 min MRT-Music)
   - Reduction in headache frequency in patients with severe radiation sickness and autonomic neuro-cerebrovascular disorders (from 93% to 12%).
   - Harmonization of autonomous innervation of cerebral arteries.
   - With slow spontaneous oscillation, function of MRT-Music as non-chemical sympatholytic.
   - Reduction of headaches in children and adults with diabetes/in older people (over 80% clients).
   - Reduction of headaches after gynecological surgery in 60% of patients.
   - Women (over 50%) with somatic disorders in the last month of pregnancy.

(2) Migraine (improvement after daily 30–40 min treatment 2–4 months)
   - Deep relaxation in 56% patients with severe migraine.

- Reduction of frequency and severity of migraine attacks in 31% patients.
- Reduction of sleep disorders in 43% of patients.
- Reduction of medication in 50% patients with severe migraine.

(3) Hormonal and immune effects

During Pregnancy (Sidorenko, 2000a)

- Improvement of hormone status in pregnant women under threat of miscarriage in the first trimester of pregnancy.
- Reduction in Cortisol by 36% in MRT-Music group, twice that of medical drug group; doubling of progesterone level, 4x as in control group; *the Kariopicnotic Index* (estradiol level dropped).
- Improvement of the hormone status in pregnant women with somatic disorders in the last month of pregnancy. Placenta-lactogen rose from 217.5 nmol/l (±5.3) to 274.9 nmol/l (±5.7) and the estriol level from 80.0 μmol/24 hours (±2) to 103.3 μmol/24 hours (±1.7), which clearly demonstrated a positive effect of the MRT-Music on the function of the fetal-placental unit and thus on the well-being of pregnant lady and fetus.
- Reduction of high hormone levels in women during parturition. Beta-endorphin value dropped by 6.05 units, ACTH showed a tendency to decrease, calming hormonal manifestations of stress.

Radiation Sickness (Sidorenko, 2000b)

Improvement in immune status in children suffering from radiation sickness

- Before treatment the immunogram of the children showed humoral disorders. Two weeks after MRT-Music the immunogram of 25% patients was normal with normalization of the AMG-factor, cellular immunity and the T- and B-lymphocytes. In the remaining 75% patients immune status improved clearly.
- Stimulation of lowered hormone levels in patients severely sick from radiation disease.
- After the 10th MRT-Music (30–40min/d) the beta-endorphin level increased by 60% to reach normal levels.
- Reduction in sleep disorders (95% down to 17% after 10 days MRT-Music).

- Improvement of the psychosomatic status of children (59% down to 23%) with reduced use of tranquilizers.

(4) Hearing Problems

- Improvement in function of hearing in 57% children with tubal disorder with negative pressure reduced by 15 mmH2O. Audiograms and impedancometry documented a clear improvement in sound-transmission capability, also subjectively confirmed by the children. In 5% of the children with conductive deafness, audiogram showed a reduced bone-air interval by 10–15 dB indicating a better hearing ability.

Apart from the common 18 types of MRT-Music, some practical examples of MRT-Music applications in other clinical fields are listed below (Chan SPJ, Chiu YK, Chui YC):

(1) Relaxation — 931,932,106 (parasympathetic); 128,935,940 (sympathetic)
(2) R&L Brain Synchrony, Autonomic Balance, Shoulder/neck pain — 1449, 941, 105 (Gynae), 279 (Golden Brain: 3 Virtuos Pianos)
(3) Severe Stress — 102 (Harmony)
(4) Pain control — 931, 942, 943
(5) Insomnia, BPH, frequency — 106, 932
(6) Peri-menopausal — 105 (Gynae), 942 (mother and child), (or 934 Preg & Child birth, 932 General Stress)
(7) 1449 (Du Mai) vs 1444 (Ren Mai)
(8) Yoga/qi-qong practitioner — Seven Chakras music
(9) Aesthetic med practitioner — twelve Meridians music
(10) TCM, counselor — 932, 921 (courage to face life), 951 (mental distress & fear)

9.1 Acupuncture and Music Therapy

Acupuncture and music therapy have both been used in various neurological and mental illnesses. The author reviewed evidence-based literature on their different clinical effects and inter-relationship with insights into proposed mechanisms of action. A systematic literature search of electronic scientific databases (English language 1989–2010 NLM/Pubmed,

Medline, Embase, PsycInfo, Google-scholars on "acupuncture and music therapy" outcomes (* RCT, systemic review) was performed. Evidence-based outcomes of acupuncture and music therapy and proposed mechanisms were explored.

Liu (2005) in a 100-day RCT of 41 Alzheimer patients found that music therapy added to acupuncture significantly improved MMSE and ADL. In a 36-week RCT of 60 cerebral palsy children, acupuncture plus music improved outcomes on motor functions. It was also demonstrated that 30 minutes music during acupuncture relieved anxiety but not enhancing pain relief (Yu *et al.*, 2009a and b). Rossignol (2009) systematically reviewed treatment of autism spectrum disorders showing Level A evidence for music therapy but only Level C evidence for acupuncture. There is no simple explanation to the differences. Liu (2010) comprehensively reviewed mechanisms of acupuncture studied in recent decade. Stimuli at acupoints and meridians (Omura, 1989 — acupuncture, electrical stimulation, mechanical stimulation, soft laser stimulation, Qi Gong; Hwang, 1992 — anatomy/class, Yung, 2004a, b and 2005 — Birdcage model) echoes important link between stimuli at dynamic acupoints/meridians and neurohormonal/cellular changes of internal organs.

Kim (2004) examined the 60s stimulatory effect of five oriental musical tones (frequency range 261.6 Hz to 440 Hz) on 20 healthy adults through headphones, skin (via speakers) and both. Greatest response of tone/organ pairs: *Gung* (261.6 Hz)/spleen, *Sang* (293.7 Hz)/lung, *Gak* (329.6 Hz)/liver, *Chi* (392.0 Hz)/heart, *Wu* (440.0 Hz)/kidney (findings consistent with traditional descriptions of Yellow Emperor Nei-Jing) suggests certain *vibration* frequencies activate certain meridians/internal organs.

9.2 Specific Acupoints and Meridians

In contrast, Zhao (2006) stimulated specific acupoint Yintang (EX-HN 3) during singing — expanding and unifying of vocal range of the singer and strengthening vocal function (coordination and completeness). Wei (2007) demonstrated in 34 normal subjects the gender differences and specific receiving sensibilities of music wave vibration at different acupoints on the hand's six channels using a radiating/receiving sound wave system; Vibromusic vibration wave total receiving music sound power (RMS) was measured at different acupoints on hand's six channels versus non-acupuncture showed gender differences (RMS at Daling (PC 7) and Shaohai (HT 3) (female > male) and specific receiving sensibility of Taiyuan (LU 9) versus other acupoints. Bratila (2007) found that harmonic sounds 124 Hz and 120 Hz excited the Lung and Kidney Meridians respectively, suggesting that acupoints have resonant vibration frequency through which an informational resonance phenomenon passed through meridians and internal organs to restore body rhythm and well-being. The original method applied measurement and electronic sound stimulation at Meridian Entry Point, measurement at Meridian Exit Point, computer data processing and biofeedback adjustment of music stimulation parameters. The outcomes showed that acupuncture stimulation among females was 7% more intense than males. In 87% cases, mean 124 Hz (122–128 Hz) excited Lung (LU) Meridian, *Shoutaiyin Feijing*. In 67% cases, mean 120 Hz (118–121 Hz) excited Kidney (KI) Meridian, *Zushaoyin Shenjing*. The author suggests that (1) acupoints have resonant "vibration frequency signature" through which an informational resonance phenomenon passed through meridians and internal organs to restore body rhythm and well-being, and (2) harmonic generation, electronic excitation, low excitation status of acupuncture points was considered a resonance phenomenon. Wang (2009) supported this harmonic vibration hypothesis by showing that acupuncture produced infrasound (2–15 Hz) at acupoints that passed through meridians easily or inducing resonance in human body directly.

Actually infrasound is observed in nature; the crocodile uses its body to generate infrasound for communication. Huge wind instruments in churches also generate infrasound that penetrates the body with potential impact on psycho-emotional state. MRT-Music is the special music therapy giving out an infrasound as low as 0.034 Hz.

Acupuncture and music therapy is thus synergistic and music helps particularly mental and psycho-emotional disorders. Insights from infrasound generation and resonant vibrations shed light on how acupuncture may work and how special Medical Resonance Therapy Music® (audible to 0.034 Hz) may be a great adjunct to acupuncture through a common pathway for various stimuli at acupoints and effects on meridian system.

9.3 Conclusion

Medical Resonance Therapy Music® should not be overlooked as its new developments have already expanded from Western medicine applications (18 types RRR CDs) to Chinese medicine (music of different Meridians), chiropractic practice (dragon music for spine health), ayurvedic Medicine (music of Chakras energy centers), mindfulness based meditation (music of meditation) and education (whole brain nurture, creativity and intelligence).

The strength of Western Medicine lies in cure of infectious diseases, surgeries and emergency life saving. Chinese Medicine is strong in managing sub-health before diseases emerge. Natural Medicine goes back to basics of nature and adopts our self-healing power to promote health. However, Medical Resonance Therapy Music® should be considered as a complementary therapy of health problems, but not replacing evidence-based Western Medicines.

References

Brătilă, F. and Moldovan, C. (2007) Music acupuncture stimulation method. *Rom J. Intern. Med.* **45**(4), 407–411.

Chiu, Y.K. (eds.) (2003) *Awakening Your Universe: The Power of Micro Music I*, 1st Ed. Natural Life Publishing Co., Taipei, pp. 20–222.

Chiu, Y.K. (eds.) (2005) *Eastern Music Treatment*, 1st Ed. Bai Sin Book Co., Taipei, pp. 94–137.

Chui, Y.C. and Hui, K.K. (2003) *Regain Inner Natural Harmonic Rhythm — The Best Prescription for Modern Man with Mind-Body Imbalance,* 1st Ed. Shui Sing Cultural Publishing Co., Taiwan, pp. 57–86.

Hwang, Y.C. (1992) Anatomy and classification of acupoints. *Probl. Vet. Med.* **4**(1), 12–15.

Kim, Y.C., Jeong, D.M. and Lee, M.S. (2004) An examination of the relationship between five oriental musical tones and corresponding internal organs and meridians. *Acupunct. Electrother. Res.* **29**(3–4), 227–233.

Koelsch, S., Fritz, T., Schulze, K., Alsop, D. and Schlaug, G. (2005) Adults and children processing music: an fMRI study. *Neuroimage* **25**(4), 1068–1076.

Lazaroff, I. and Shimshoni, R. (2000) Effects of Medical Resonance Therapy Music on patients with psoriasis and neurodermatitis — a pilot study. *Integr. Physiol. Behav. Sci.* **35**(3), 189–198.

Lee, Y.K. (eds.) (2000) *Listen and Smile with Energy — the Miraculous Medical Resonance Therapy Music*, 1st Ed. Natural Life Publishing Co., Taipei, pp. 10–190.

Leventhall, G. (2007) What is infrasound? *Prog. Biophys. Mol. Biol.* **93**(1–3), 130–137.

Liu, G. and Yuan, L.X. (2005) Clinical observation on acupuncture combined with music for treatment of Alzheimer disease. *Zhongguo Zhen Jiu* **25**(6), 390–392.

Liu, J.L., Wang, J.Y., Chen, S.P., Gao, Y.H., Qiao, L.N. and Han, Y.J. (2010) Progress in the study on the mechanism underlying the correlation between acupoints/meridians and Zangfu organs. *Zhen Ci Yan Jiu* **35**(1), 71–77.

Nickel, A.K., Hillecke, T., Argstatter, H. and Bolay, H.V. (2005) Outcome research in music therapy: a step on the long road to an evidence-based treatment. *Ann. N. Y. Acad. Sci.* **1060**, 283–293.

Oelkers-Ax, R., Leins, A., Parzer, P., Hillecke, T., Bolay, H.V., Fischer, J., Bender, S., Hermanns, U. and Resch, F. (2008) Butterbur root extract and music therapy in the prevention of childhood migraine: an explorative study. *Eur. J. Pain* **12**(3), 301–313.

Omura, Y. (1989) Connections found between each meridian (heart, stomach, triple burner, etc.) and organ representation area of corresponding internal organs in each side of the cerebral cortex; release of common neurotransmitters and hormones unique to each meridian and corresponding acupuncture point and internal organ after acupuncture, electrical stimulation, mechanical stimulation (including shiatsu), soft laser stimulation or qi gong. *Acupunct. Electrother. Res.* **14**(2), 155–186.

Rossignol, D.A. (2009) Novel and emerging treatments for autism spectrum disorders: a systematic review. *Ann. Clin. Psychiatry* **21**(4), 213–236.

Shemagonov, A.V. and Sidorenko, V.N. (2000) Can the Medical Resonance Therapy Music affect autonomous innervation of cerebral arteries? *Integr. Physiol. Behav. Sci.* **35**(3), 218–223.

Sidorenko, V.N. (2000a) Clinical application of Medical Resonance Therapy Music in high-risk pregnancies. *Integr. Physiol. Behav. Sci.* **35**(3), 199–207.

Sidorenko, V.N. (2000b) Effects of the Medical Resonance Therapy Music on haemodynamic parameter in children with autonomic nervous system disturbances. *Integr. Physiol. Behav. Sci.* **35**(3), 208–211.

Sidorenko, V.N. (2000c) Effects of the Medical Resonance Therapy Music in the complex treatment of epileptic patients. *Integr. Physiol. Behav. Sci.* **35**(3), 212–217.

Trappe, H.J. (2009) Music and health — what kind of music is helpful for whom? What music not? *Dtsch. Med. Wochenschr.* **134**(51–52), 2601–2606.

Wang, X.M. (2009) Analysis on the mechanism of acupuncture infrasound energy in treatment of diseases. *Zhongguo Zhen Jiu* **29**(3), 223–226.

Wang, X.M. (2011) Lifting-thrusting and rotating manipulations: a comparison on energy input. *Zhongguo Zhen Jiu* **31**(1), 71–74.

Wei, Y.L., Yang, Y., Tu, Y.W., Kong, J., Han, B., Liu, G.L. and Liu, W. (2007) Observation on the receiving sensibilities of the points on the hand's six channels for vibromusic sound wave. *Zhongguo Zhen Jiu* **27**(4), 269–272.

Yu, H., Liu, Y., Li, S. and Ma, X. (2009a) Effects of music on anxiety and pain in children with cerebral palsy receiving acupuncture: a randomized controlled trial. *Int. J. Nurs. Stud.* **46**(11), 1423–1430.

Yu, H.B., Liu, Y.F. and Wu, L.X. (2009b) Acupuncture combined with music therapy for treatment of 30 cases of cerebral palsy. *J. Tradit. Chin. Med.* **29**(4), 243–248.

Yung, K.T. (2004a) A birdcage model for the Chinese Meridian System: part I. A channel as a transmission line. *Am. J. Chin. Med.* **32**(5), 815–828.

Yung, K.T. (2004b) A birdcage model for the Chinese meridian system: part II. The meridian system as a birdcage resonator. *Am. J. Chin. Med.* **32**(6), 985–997.

Yung, K.T. (2005) Birdcage model for the Chinese meridian system: part VI. meridians as the primary regulatory system. *Am. J. Chin. Med.* **33**(5), 759–766.

Zhao, L. (2006) Observation on stimulation of yintang (EX-HN 3) promoting the action of expanding and unifying the vocal range of the singer. *Zhongguo Zhen Jiu* **26**(5), 343–345.

Chapter 10

Neuroscience and Meditation

Tatia M. C. Lee, Nerissa S. P. Ho, Jing Yin, Chack-Fan Lee
Chetwyn C. H. Chan and Kwok-Fai So

Abstract

Meditation is a family of practices that cultivate specific psychological states or mental capacities for heightened self-awareness and insight. Neuroscientists have found that regular and sustained meditation has significant structural and functional effects on the brain. Structural and functional neuroimaging have linked meditation to improved regulation of the default network of attention, controlled focus, and sustained attention. Studies have also linked meditation practice with the cultivation of positive emotion. In part because of the evidence that it causes neurobiological changes, support is growing for research on the potential use of meditation for therapies promoting cognitive and affective processing, which should ultimately lift physiological and psychological well-being. Thus far, research outcomes are largely positive and only rarely accompanied by adverse side effects, suggesting that meditation is a promising therapy — and may even help prevent some psychopathologies. Future research should continue to examine the potential healing and restorative effects of meditation.

Keywords: Meditation; Neuroplasticity; Attention; Positive Emotion.

Meditation is a family of practices aimed at cultivating specific psychological states or mental capacities, such as mindfulness, equanimity, wisdom, or compassion (Salzberg, 1995; Lutz *et al.*, 2008b). Meditation is a long-standing tradition in Asian and other cultures. It is not a religion itself and has been increasingly practiced by people without any religious affiliations, such as in modern yoga, Tai Chi, and QiGong. It has also been applied in mindfulness interventions (Kabat-Zinn, 2003).

There are different styles and traditions of meditative practice. Some of the leading styles include focused-attention meditation, open-monitoring meditation; and loving-kindness meditation (Salzberg, 1995; Lutz *et al.*, 2008b). Despite the diverse styles of practice, meditation commonly emphasizes the cultivation of awareness and insight, leading to the state of meditative quiescence and equanimity (Houshmand *et al.*, 2002).

Quiescence is to be tranquility at rest — a completely relaxed bodily state with full concentration on the present moment. This allows the meditator to achieve intense mental focus, attentional stability, and attentional clarity without going astray for a very long time (Houshmand *et al.*, 2002).

Meditative equanimity, on the other hand, is the insight to accept things as they are, with a balanced state of mind that is calm and spacious. This enables one to be present, fully and non-judgmentally. This lets people experience the fact that circumstances are perpetually changing. The end state is a state of dispassion, endowing loving kindness, compassion, and sympathetic joy (Salzberg, 1995).

10.1 Neuroplasticity

What has neuroscience discovered about meditation? To explore this question, let us first look at the concept of neuroplasticity. Neuroscientists have discovered that human brains are malleable and susceptible to alterations in response to the demands of environmental stimulations (Maguire *et al.*, 2000; Munte *et al.*, 2002). Researchers believe that these changes happen in response to changing demands and are confined to the areas involved in specific kinds of processing (Draganski *et al.*, 2004).

Neuroplasticity is a fundamental mechanism for neuronal adaptation that can happen at different levels of the brain. At the structural level, there can be morphological changes in the spines and dendrites — even new neuron growth in adult brains (adult neurogenesis). At the functional level, there can be synaptic plasticity that affects neural circuitry operations and synaptic transmission for long-term potentiation, including the generation of new synapses (synaptogenesis). Neuroplasticity may also involve molecular changes, especially molecules of neurotransmission and their receptor cells. It may affect the molecules that transmit signals at the synapses. Finally, neuroplasticity may work through cells, by introducing new genes and causing the production of new proteins (Pittenger and Duman, 2007; Sanes and Lichtman, 1999).

People generally think that neuroplasticity is beneficial to brain functioning (Pittenger and Duman, 2007; Mesulam, 1999; Manji *et al.*, 2000). Scientists have speculated that neuroplasticity could help protect people against cognitive decline during aging. It may also help people restore functioning after injuries to the central nervous system (Kempermann *et al.*, 2002; Rojas Vega *et al.*, 2008; Mahncke *et al.*, 2006).

Nonetheless, neuroplasticity can sometimes be maladaptive. Past studies have found that abnormal neuroplasticity was associated with focal dystonia, sometimes known as musicians' cramp, which seems to be caused by degradation of cortical representation and dedifferentiation of sensory feedback information (Elbert *et al.*, 1998; Quartarone and Pisani, 2011). These mechanisms were also responsible for dyskinesia, a complication during dopamine-mimetic treatment of Parkinson's disease (Cenci, 2007).

Fascinated by the exceptional mental states achievable with meditative quiescence and equanimity, neuroscientists started studying how meditation changes the human brain (Houshmand *et al.*, 2002; Davidson, 2005). Results from their studies shed light on the neural underpinnings of the key psychological processes in cognition and emotion, and they opened the doorway for people to use meditation as an alternative way to treat mental disorders.

Researchers and clinical practitioners have shown that cultivating the sorts of mental capacities associated with meditation can restore homeostasis and promote psychological health. This resembles Chinese medicine's focus on physical and mental health through balancing *yin* and *yang* (the mind-body harmony). Hence, meditation is sometimes being regarded as an alternative method for health training and therapy. In brief, researchers have proposed that regular and sustained practice of meditation is an environmental stimulation for neuroplasticity. This postulation fits well with meditative teachings, especially with their emphasis on cultivating durable trait changes in quiescence, equanimity, and compassion.

To dig deeper into the relationship between meditation and neuroplasticity, neuroscientists have started using neurophysiological and neuroimaging techniques, such as electroencephalography (EEG) and functional magnetic resonance imaging (fMRI). These techniques may help explain the long-term trait changes associated with experience-induced brain changes.

The ultimate goal is to shed light on the potential clinical values of meditation for promoting cognitive and affective functioning, as well as well-being.

10.2 Structural Anatomical Changes of the Brain

Evidence that meditation brings about anatomical changes in brain structures is abundant. Meditators have increased cortical thickness and gray matter concentration in regions associated with attention, interoceptive awareness, and sensory processing, including the prefrontal cortex and right anterior insula. These structural differences correlate with the amount of meditation experience (Lazar et al., 2005; Hölzel *et al.*, 2008). Other researchers have suggested that regular meditation would help shield the brain from normal aging, in terms of both sustained attention and gray matter volume (Pagnoni and Cekic, 2007).

Meditators also have significantly dense gray matter in the right orbitofrontal cortex (Luders *et al.*, 2009) and right hippocampus (Luders *et al.*, 2009; Leung *et al.*, 2013). The researchers proposed that these areas are related to enhanced emotional regulation and response control, which are both associated with meditation.

There is also evidence that meditation causes structural reorganization of the brain along affective processing pathways. Meditators have been found to have thicker cortices in the dorsal anterior cingulate and the bilateral secondary somatosensory cortex. They also have more gray matter in the anterior cingulate and certain primary somatosensory cortex areas — both of which correlated with hours of meditation experience. Cortical thickness of these brain regions were found to correlate negatively with pain sensitivity (Grant *et al.*, 2010).

Another brain region that experienced meditators have dense gray matter is the lower brainstem region. This finding led researchers to postulate that meditation improves cardiorespiratory control and immunoreactivity, in addition to its more well-known cognitive and emotional effects (Vestergaard-Poulsen *et al.*, 2009).

10.3 Functional Changes in the Brain

Previous findings have suggested that meditators have exceptional attentional focus that they can sustain over a very long time without distraction. They also have more positive emotions even in the face of difficult situations. Based on these findings, many meditation studies have focused on positive emotion and attention (e.g. Lee *et al.*, 2012). To test these outcomes scientifically, researchers have (1) measured differences between experienced and non-experienced meditators; (2) watched meditators' neural responses between baseline (non-meditative) and meditation; (3) tested for long-term trait changes in behavioral tests comparing long-term meditators, novices, and non-meditators; and (4) more directly tested the causality of meditation by conducting longitudinal studies comparing the same group of meditators before and after training.

10.3.1 *Attention*

Attention is one of the most crucial concepts in cognition, from basic consciousness to memory and learning. Meditation and attention are closely linked; meditation directly trains concentration, focusing consciousness on the present moment. Meditation requires practitioners to exert their executive system to control attention (Raz and Buhle, 2006; Posner, 1994). In fact, the same regions that activate when people enter into meditation are the regions that show abnormalities in people with attention deficit disorders (Brefczynski-Lewis *et al.*, 2007).

10.3.1.1 *Regulation of the default mode network (DMN)*

The DMN engineers an automatic cascade of semantic associations in response to external stimuli based on conditioned thoughts and previously acquired feelings and behaviors (Pagnoni *et al.*, 2008). The level of activity of the DMN is inversely related to cognitive load: when cognitive load is low, the DMN is active (Raichle and Snyder, 2007). This pattern of activity suggests that the human brain is implicitly biased towards DMN processing. The DMN is also active during self-referential mental activity (Kelley *et al.*, 2002). Unless it is being consciously controlled, the brain can be distracted from effortful attention. Regulation of the DMN refers to the cognitive effort and ability that keep the mind from wandering into processing spontaneous neuronal activities (Fox and Raichle, 2007). Previous empirical studies have shown that meditation lessens Stroop interference, implying that it voluntarily reduces habitual processing (Heidi, 2005).

Pagnoni and colleagues (2008) reported that experienced meditators are better at regulating spontaneous mental activities, resulting in reduced post-stimulus tail and better re-focusing during a lexical decision task that was interspersed with simplified meditation. Furthermore, studies of the DMN have found different results based on different forms of meditation. For example, an EEG study reported that practice of transcendental meditation was associated with higher power and coherence for alpha1 brain waves in regions that overlap with the DMN — frontal areas, rather than lateral areas (Travis *et al.*, 2010). On the other hand, an fMRI study found that long-term practitioners of focused-attention meditation had *less* activation in regions associated with the DMN when distracters were presented to interfere the meditation (Brefczynski-Lewis *et al.*, 2007).

Some researchers have proposed that training in mindfulness meditation could help dissociate the self-referential network (which focuses on self experiences extended across time, characterized by midline cortical activation) from the habitual linguistic-semantic network (left lateralized network). Instead, meditation may encourage people to engage their self-referential network that focuses on the momentary self and experiences the present moment (Farb *et al.*, 2007).

10.3.1.2 *Sustained attention*

A considerable number of behavioral studies have provided evidence for the link between meditation practice and attention-control skills. Compared to non-meditators, practitioners of both focused-attention and open-monitoring meditation were found to be less susceptible to Stroop interference, although not global-local letters task interference (Wang *et al.*, 2005). The authors suggested that these meditation practices enhance attention focus for competitive selection by monitoring conflicts from sensory inputs and inhibiting prepotent responses, rather than filtering out salient stimuli.

Parallel with this finding, focused-attention meditation seems to promote selective-attention stability as measured by a reduction in the variability of reaction times and neural responses while discerning auditory stimuli (Lutz *et al.*, 2009). Similarly, a longitudinal study compared pre- and post-training performances and found that meditation enhanced perceptual sensitivity toward sensory information (MacLean *et al.*, 2010). This led to a reduction in the amount of resources used for attention discrimination and improvement in the vigilance of sustained attention.

Neuroimaging studies have given further evidence of the potential effect of meditation on neural mechanisms associated with attention. An EEG study found that long-term meditators have more gamma oscillations (25–42 Hz) than slow rhythms (4–13 Hz), as well as increased phase synchrony of gamma waves across widely separated regions of the brain, compared to non-meditators (Lutz *et al.*, 2004). The differences even held when they compared meditators in a non-meditative state with non-meditators. Furthermore, the group differences increased during meditation and lasted into the post-meditative state (Melloni *et al.*, 2007).

Furthermore, focused attention during meditation also increased the phase consistency of theta-band (3–7 Hz) neural oscillation in response to target stimuli (Lutz *et al.*, 2009). As claimed by the authors, these neural responses reflected the increased cortical signal-to-noise ratio in the neural network for sustained attention, allowing heightened cognitive control for inhibiting distracters.

Researchers have proposed that meditation does not immediately reduce the activity required for attention (Brefczynski-Lewis *et al.*, 2007; Lutz *et al.*, 2009). Initially, meditation actually seems to increase activation in the attention network, particularly in areas associated with sustained attention. Only after extensive practice does activation in those areas decrease. That produces an inverted u-shaped learning curve, which is similar to the pattern of the acquisition of other skills. It was postulated that this learning curve reflected the way that meditation could promote neuroplasticity in order to improve the efficiency of cortical activity — eventually letting meditators sustain attention with less cognitive effort.

10.3.2 *Positive emotion*

Loving-kindness meditation (LKM) emphasizes the wish for happiness and the cultivation of compassion. However, the meaning of happiness for loving-kindness meditators is different from its ordinary sense. Most people think of happiness as experiencing pleasure and satisfaction or as being free from pain and suffering. Loving-kindness meditators believe the quest for this kind of happiness is delusive. Instead, they believe that happiness stems from the insight of equanimity. They believe that, through our complete and genuine presence of mind, we can accept our true nature and integrate all aspects of our experiences with everyone and everything, and then experience love and compassion.

Meditation's potential to foster positive emotions and reduce negative ones has inspired neuroscientists to study its effect on affective processing. For positive emotions, focused-attention meditation seems to cause emotionally positive "blissful" experiences (Aftanas and Golocheikine, 2001). Similarly, regular practice of LKM increased the daily experiences of positive emotions that should build up personal resources for increased life satisfaction (Fredrickson *et al.*, 2008).

Researchers have made some progress in understanding how meditation promotes positive emotions. Using high-resolution EEG to measure neural oscillations, researchers reported that the emotionally positive "blissful" experience of long-term meditators corresponded to increased theta synchronization in the anterior frontal and midline regions, as well as enhanced long-connectivity of theta oscillations between the prefrontal and posterior association cortex (Aftanas and Golocheikine, 2001).

Moreover, functional imaging results suggested that voluntarily generating compassion during LKM helped to cultivate concern for others, especially in response to others' negative emotions. Loving-kindness meditators showed increased neural activations in brain areas associated with emotion sharing and perspective taking. Furthermore, the strength of activation correlated with the self-reported intensity of meditation (Lutz *et al.*, 2008a). Functional imaging also found that meditation could increase left-sided activation in anterior regions associated with positive emotions (Davidson *et al.*, 2003).

Of negative emotions, pain is the most frequently studied feeling in meditation research. Researchers have proposed several mechanisms by which meditation might be able to reduce pain: by distracting attention away from the source of pain, by decreasing the physiological response to pain, by lowering anxiety and stress associated with pain anticipation, and by reducing pain-related distress. Each of these mechanisms might be exerted to different degrees by different styles of meditation (Orme-Johnson *et al.*, 2006).

Some studies have found that practitioners of both focused-attention and open-monitoring meditation experience the same level of pain intensity as non-meditators when exposed to painful stimuli. However, the pain distressed the practitioners of open-monitoring meditation less, suggesting that meditation affects the cognitive evaluation of pain, rather than the sensory experience (Orme-Johnson *et al.*, 2006; Perlman *et al.*, 2010; Mills and Farrow, 1981). Another study reported that mindfulness meditation reduced pain by reducing pain sensitivity (Zeidan *et al.*, 2010).

Furthermore, meditators have shown weaker activity in the thalamus, the secondary somatosensory cortex (insula), and cingulate cortex during meditation, which might be related to the emotional aspects of lower pain perception (Kakigi *et al.*, 2005). Furthermore, researchers proposed that the affect-labeling technique that meditators use was the neurocognitive mechanism for reducing negative affect. Their key piece of evidence was that affect labeling was associated with a neural activation pattern that was more widespread in the prefrontal cortex, but reduced in the bilateral amygdala (a brain region associated with negative emotion). This sort of activation pattern was positively correlated with the level of dispositional mindfulness (Creswell *et al.*, 2007).

10.4 Potential Therapeutic Value of Meditation

With the existing neurobiological evidence of meditation's beneficial effect on brain anatomy — both structurally and functionally — there has been increasing support for testing meditation's usefulness in therapy. Meditation may be able to improve physiological and psychological well-being (Morone *et al.*, 2008; Mansky and Wallerstedt, 2006). To date, results from many of these clinical applications have suggested positive clinical outcomes, with rare adverse effects (Arias *et al.*, 2006).

One of the most widespread clinical applications of meditation therapy is to reduce stress or anxiety; this is the goal of mindfulness-based stress reduction (MBSR; Kabat-Zinn *et al.*, 1998) and integrative body-mind training (Tang *et al.*, 2007). Some have argued that the clinical effectiveness of mindfulness meditation is really just due to the psychosocial confounds of meditation, since most MBSRs train people in groups (although individual therapy is also possible, for example, with audiotaped instructions (Kabat-Zinn, 2003). Future studies will still need to better control for the potential group effect.

However, it is certainly plausible that the therapeutic effect comes from the bodily relaxation technique of mindfulness training. Relaxation may encourage participants to develop the mental flexibility needed to better tolerate stressful experiences. This differs from classical psychotherapy, which emphasizes covert coping strategies to eliminate or avoid threats. The results so far have been encouraging, reducing both self-ratings and therapists' ratings of anxiety and panic symptoms. There have also been improvements in stress-related physiological reactivity, such as lowered levels of cortisol, better immune functioning, and anti-inflammatory response (Davidson *et al.*, 2003; Tang *et al.*, 2007; Carlson *et al.*, 2003; Kabat-Zinn *et al.*, 1992; MacLean *et al.*, 1997). These findings suggest that meditation could reduce rates of disease from viral infections or other pathogens. Studies have also found that meditation improves sleep quality, with less disruption from fatigue and mood disturbances (Carlson and Garland, 2005; Williams *et al.*, 2005).

Meditation has also been used in interventions for depression (Ramel *et al.*, 2004; Mason and Hargreaves, 2001), chronic pain (Kabat-Zinn, 1982; Kabat-Zinn *et al.*, 1985), and grieving (Sagula and Rice, 2004). The idea is that meditation training helps people control affective processing and emotional reactivity. This, in turn, may help people reduce rumination and catastrophizing, which magnify negative effects.

Because meditation trains people in awareness and self-regulation strategies, it may be useful in treating psychopathological disorders. For example, researchers have proposed that meditation might help treat and prevent relapse of addictive behaviours, including substance and alcohol abuse, pathological gambling, and compulsive eating (Marlatt, 2002; Zgierska *et al.*, 2008; Bowen *et al.*, 2006; Kristeller and Hallett, 1999; de Lisle *et al.*, 2011). Some researchers proposed displacing people's "negative addiction" to substances with a "positive addiction" to meditation (Marlatt and Chawla, 2007).

As yet another example, meditation has been used as an adjunctive therapy for social and communication disorders, including schizophrenia and attention-deficit-hyperactivity disorder (ADHD; Zylowska *et al.*, 2008;

Johnson *et al.*, 2011). The pilot results of these early studies are promising for meditation therapy to become an intervention for the treatment and prevention of psychopathological disorders.

10.5 Conclusions

To date, the findings of meditation on neuroplasticity have been encouraging. There is promise in meditation's application toward promoting cognitive (attention) and affective processing (positive emotion). Future neuroscientific studies may further our understanding of the neural basis of meditation by looking at (1) the different forms of meditation practice, (2) the quality and intensity of practice, and (3) individual differences in incorporating meditation skills into everyday experiences. Studies also need to control for other potential confounding factors, which include environmental factors in meditation practice, psychosocial factors from the influence of the teachers and the supportive practicing group, and the self-selection effect of long-term meditation.

In sum, preliminary neurobiological evidence for the effect of meditation on positive neuroplasticity has provided a solid base for the therapeutic application of meditation to improve physical and psychological well-being. And while the underlying neural mechanisms are still not fully understood, the preliminary evidence also supports meditation as a potential adjunctive therapy for psychopathological disorders. The gold standard of interventions — randomized controlled clinical trials — for meditation therapy are not far away, if not already underway.

Acknowledgment

This work was supported by the Research Grant Council General Research Fund [HKU747612H] to T. Lee.

References

Aftanas, L.I. and Golocheikine, S.A. (2001) Human anterior and frontal midline theta and lower alpha reflect emotionally positive state and internalized attention: high-resolution EEG investigation of meditation. *Neurosci. Lett.* **310**, 57–60.

Arias, A.J., Steinberg, K., Banga, A. and Trestman, R.L. (2006) Systematic review of the efficacy of meditation techniques as treatments for medical illness. *J. Altern. Complement. Med.* **12**, 817–832.

Bowen, S., Witkiewitz, K., Dillworth, T.M., Chawla, N., Simpson, T.L., Ostafin, B.D., Larimer, M.E., Blume, A.W., Parks, G.A. and Marlatt, G.A. (2006) Mindfulness meditation and substance use in an incarcerated population. *Psychol. Addict. Behav.* **20**, 343–347.

Brefczynski-Lewis, J.A., Lutz, A., Schaefer, H.S., Levinson, D.B. and Davidson, R.J. (2007) Neural correlates of attentional expertise in long-term meditation practitioners. *Proc. Natl. Acad. Sci. USA* **104**, 11483–11488.

Carlson, L.E., Speca, M., Patel, K.D. and Goodey, E. (2003) Mindfulness-based stress reduction in relation to quality of life, mood, symptoms of stress, and immune parameters in breast and prostate cancer outpatients. *Psychosom. Med.* **65**, 571–581.

Carlson, L. and Garland, S. (2005) Impact of mindfulness-based stress reduction (MBSR) on sleep, mood, stress and fatigue symptoms in cancer outpatients. *Int. J. Behav. Med.* **12**, 278–285.

Cenci, M.A. (2007) Dopamine dysregulation of movement control in l-DOPA-induced dyskinesia. *Trends. Neurosci.* **30**, 236–243.

Creswell, J.D., Way, B.M., Eisenberger, N.I. and Lieberman, M.D. (2007) Neural correlates of dispositional mindfulness during affect labeling. *Psychosom. Med.* **69**, 560–565.

Davidson, R.J., Kabat-Zinn, J., Schumacher, J., Rosenkranz, M., Muller, D., Santorelli, S.F., Urbanowski, F., Harrington, A., Bonus, K. and Sheridan, J.F. (2003) Alterations in brain and immune function produced by mindfulness meditation. *Psychosom. Med.* **65**, 564–570.

Davidson, R.J. (2005) Meditation and neuroplasticity: training your brain. *Explore (NY)* **1**, 380–388.

de Lisle, S.M., Dowling, N.A. and Sabura Allen, J. (2011) Mindfulness-based cognitive therapy for problem gambling. *Clin. Case Studies* **10**, 210–228.

Draganski, B., Gaser, C., Busch, V., Schuierer, G., Bogdahn, U. and May, A. (2004) Neuroplasticity: changes in grey matter induced by training. *Nature* **427**, 311–312.

Elbert, T., Candia, V., Altenmuller, E., Rau, H., Sterr, A., Rockstroh, B., Pantev, C. and Taub, E. (1998) Alteration of digital representations in somatosensory cortex in focal hand dystonia. *Neuroreport* **9**, 3571–3575.

Farb, N.A., Segal, Z.V., Mayberg, H., Bean, J., McKeon, D., Fatima, Z. and Anderson, A.K. (2007) Attending to the present: mindfulness meditation reveals distinct neural modes of self-reference. *Soc. Cogn. Affect. Neurosci.* **2**, 313–322.

Fox, M.D. and Raichle, M.E. (2007) Spontaneous fluctuations in brain activity observed with functional magnetic resonance imaging. *Nat. Rev. Neurosci.* **8**, 700–711.

Fredrickson, B.L., Cohn, M.A., Coffey, K.A., Pek, J. and Finkel, S.M. (2008) Open hearts build lives: positive emotions, induced through loving-kindness meditation, build consequential personal resources. *J. Pers. Soc. Psychol.* **95**, 1045–1062.

Grant, J.A., Courtemanche, J., Duerden, E.G., Duncan, G.H. and Rainville, P. (2010) Cortical thickness and pain sensitivity in Zen meditators. *Emotion* **10**, 43–53.

Heidi, W.-S. (2005) Meditation can reduce habitual responding. *Altern. Ther. Health Med.* **11**, 42.

Hölzel, B.K., Ott, U., Gard, T., Hempel, H., Weygandt, M., Morgen, K. and Vaitl, D. (2008) Investigation of mindfulness meditation practitioners with voxel-based morphometry. *Soc. Cogn. Affect. Neurosci.* **3**, 55–61.

Houshmand, Z., Harrington, A., Saron, C. and Davidson, R.J. (2002) Training the mind: first steps in a cross-cultural collaboration in neuroscientific research. In: *Visions of Compassion: Western Scientists and Tibetan Buddhists Examine Human Nature* (eds.) Davidson, R.J. and Harrington, A. Oxford University Press, Oxford, pp. 3–17.

Johnson, D.P., Penn, D.L., Fredrickson, B.L., Kring, A.M., Meyer, P.S., Catalino, L.I. and Brantley, M. (2011) A pilot study of loving-kindness meditation for the negative symptoms of schizophrenia. *Schizophr. Res.* **129**, 137–140.

Kabat-Zinn, J. (1982) An outpatient program in behavioral medicine for chronic pain patients based on the practice of mindfulness meditation: theoretical considerations and preliminary results. *Gen. Hosp. Psychiatry* **4**, 33–47.

Kabat-Zinn, J., Lipworth, L. and Burney, R. (1985) The clinical use of mindfulness meditation for the self-regulation of chronic pain. *J. Behav. Med.* **8**, 163–190.

Kabat-Zinn, J., Massion, A.O., Kristeller, J., Peterson, L.G., Fletcher, K.E., Pbert, L., Lenderking, W.R. and Santorelli, S.F. (1992) Effectiveness of a meditation-based stress reduction program. *Am. J. Psychiatry* **149**, 936.

Kabat-Zinn, J., Wheeler, E., Light, T., Skillings, A., Scharf, M., Cropley, T., Hosmer, D. and Bernhard, J. (1998) Influence of a mindfulness meditation-based stress reduction intervention on rates of skin clearing in patients with moderate to severe psoriasis undergoing phototherapy (UVB) and photochemotherapy (PUVA). *Psychosom. Med.* **60**, 625–632.

Kabat-Zinn, J. (2003) Mindfulness-based interventions in context: past, present and future. *Clin. Psychol. Sci. Pract.* **10**, 144–156.

Kakigi, R., Nakata, H., Inui, K., Hiroe, N., Nagata, O., Honda, M., Tanaka, S., Sadato, N. and Kawakami, M. (2005) Intracerebral pain processing in a yoga master who claims not to feel pain during meditation. *Eur. J. Pain* **9**, 581–589.

Kelley, W.M., Macrae, C.N., Wyland, C.L., Caglar, S., Inati, S. and Heatherton, T.F. (2002) Finding the self? An event-related fMRI study. *J. Cogn. Neurosci.* **14**, 785–794.

Kempermann, G., Gast, D. and Gage, F.H. (2002) Neuroplasticity in old age: sustained fivefold induction of hippocampal neurogenesis by long-term environmental enrichment. *Ann. Neurol.* **52**, 135–143.

Kristeller, J.L. and Hallett, C.B. (1999) An exploratory study of a meditation-based intervention for binge eating disorder. *J. Health Psychol.* **4**, 357–363.

Lazar, S.W., Kerr, C.E., Wasserman, R.H., Gray, J.R., Greve, D.N., Treadway, M.T., McGarvey, M., Quinn, B.T., Dusek, J.A., Benson, H., Rauch, S.L., Moore, C.I. and Fischl, B. (2005) Meditation experience is associated with increased cortical thickness. *Neuroreport* **16**, 1893–1897.

Lee, T.M.C., Leung, M.K., Hou, W.K., Tang, J.C., Yin, J., So, K.F., Lee, C.F. and Chan, C.C. (2012) Distinct neural activity associated with focused-attention meditation and loving-kindness meditation. *PLoS ONE* **7**, e40054.

Leung, M.K., Chan, C.C., Yin, J., Lee, C.F., So, K.F. and Lee, T.M.C. (2013) Increased gray-matter volume in the right angular and posterior parahippocampal gyri in loving-kindness meditators. *Soc. Cogn. Affect. Neurosci.* **8**, 34–30.

Luders, E., Toga, A.W., Lepore, N. and Gaser, C. (2009) The underlying anatomical correlates of long-term meditation: larger hippocampal and frontal volumes of gray matter. *NeuroImage* **45**, 672–678.

Lutz, A., Greischar, L.L., Rawlings, N.B., Ricard, M. and Davidson, R.J. (2004) Long-term meditators self-induce high-amplitude gamma synchrony during mental practice. *Proc. Natl. Acad. Sci. USA* **101**, 16369–16373.

Lutz, A., Brefczynski-Lewis, J., Johnstone, T. and Davidson, R.J. (2008a) Regulation of the neural circuitry of emotion by compassion meditation: effects of meditative expertise. *PLoS ONE* **3**, e1897.

Lutz, A., Slagter, H.A., Dunne, J.D. and Davidson, R.J. (2008b) Attention regulation and monitoring in meditation. *Trends. Cogn. Sci.* **12**, 163–169.

Lutz, A., Slagter, H.A., Rawlings, N.B., Francis, A.D., Greischar, L.L. and Davidson, R.J. (2009) Mental training enhances attentional stability: neural and behavioral evidence. *J. Neurosci.* **29**, 13418–13427.

MacLean, C.R.K., Walton, K.G., Wenneberg, S.R., Levitsky, D.K., Mandarino, J.P., Waziri, R., Hillis, S.L. and Schneider, R.H. (1997) Effects of the transcendental meditation program on adaptive mechanisms: changes in hormone levels and responses to stress after 4 months of practice. *Psychoneuroendocrinology* **22**, 277–295.

MacLean, K.A., Ferrer, E., Aichele, S.R., Bridwell, D.A., Zanesco, A.P., Jacobs, T.L., King, B.G., Rosenberg, E.L., Sahdra, B.K., Shaver, P.R., Wallace, B.A., Mangun, G.R. and Saron, C.D. (2010) Intensive meditation training improves perceptual discrimination and sustained attention. *Psychol. Sci.* **21**, 829–839.

Maguire, E.A., Gadian, D.G., Johnsrude, I.S., Good, C.D., Ashburner, J., Frackowiak, R.S.J. and Frith, C.D. (2000) Navigation-related structural change in the hippocampi of taxi drivers. *Proc. Natl. Acad. Sci. USA* **97**, 4398–4403.

Mahncke, H.W., Connor, B.B., Appelman, J., Ahsanuddin, O.N., Hardy, J.L., Wood, R.A., Joyce, N.M., Boniske, T., Atkins, S. and Merzenich, M.M. (2006) Memory enhancement in healthy older adults using a brain plasticity-based training program: a randomized, controlled study. *Proc. Natl. Acad. Sci. USA* **103**, 12523–12528.

Manji, H.K., Moore, G.J., Rajkowska, G. and Chen, G. (2000) Neuroplasticity and cellular resilience in mood disorders. *Mol. Psychiatry* **5**, 567.

Mansky, P.J. and Wallerstedt, D.B. (2006) Complementary medicine in palliative care and cancer symptom management. *Cancer J.* **12**, 425–431.

Marlatt, G.A. (2002) Buddhist philosophy and the treatment of addictive behavior. *Cogn. Behav. Pract.* **9**, 44–50.

Marlatt, G.A. and Chawla, N. (2007) Meditation and alcohol use. *South. Med. J.* **100**, 451–453.

Mason, O. and Hargreaves, I. (2001) A qualitative study of mindfulness-based cognitive therapy for depression. *Psychol. Psychother.* **74**, 197.

Melloni, L., Molina, C., Pena, M., Torres, D., Singer, W. and Rodriguez, E. (2007) Synchronization of neural activity across cortical areas correlates with conscious perception. *J. Neurosci.* **27**, 2858–2865.

Mesulam, M.M. (1999) Neuroplasticity failure in Alzheimer's disease: bridging the gap between plaques and tangles. *Neuron* **24**, 521–529.

Mills, W.W. and Farrow, J.T. (1981) The transcendental meditation technique and acute experimental pain. *Psychosom. Med.* **43**, 157–164.

Morone, N.E., Greco, C.M. and Weiner, D.K. (2008) Mindfulness meditation for the treatment of chronic low back pain in older adults: a randomized controlled pilot study. *Pain.* **134**, 310–319.

Munte, T.F., Altenmuller, E. and Jancke, L. (2002) The musician's brain as a model of neuroplasticity. *Nat. Rev. Neurosci.* **3**, 473–478.

Orme-Johnson, D.W., Schneider, R.H., Son, Y.D., Nidich, S. and Cho, Z-H. (2006) Neuroimaging of meditation's effect on brain reactivity to pain. *Neuroreport* **17**, 1359–1363.

Pagnoni, G. and Cekic, M. (2007) Age effects on gray matter volume and attentional performance in Zen meditation. *Neurobiol. Aging* **28**, 1623–1627.

Pagnoni, G., Cekic, M. and Guo, Y. (2008) "Thinking about not-thinking": neural correlates of conceptual processing during Zen meditation. *PLoS ONE* **3**, e3083.

Perlman, D.M., Salomons, T.V., Davidson, R.J. and Lutz, A. (2010) Differential effects on pain intensity and unpleasantness of two meditation practices. *Emotion* **10**, 65–71.

Pittenger, C. and Duman, R.S. (2007) Stress, depression, and neuroplasticity: a convergence of mechanisms. *Neuropsychopharmacology* **33**, 88–109.

Posner, M.I. (1994) Attention: the mechanisms of consciousness. *Proc. Natl. Acad. Sci. USA* **91**, 7398–7403.

Quartarone, A. and Pisani, A. (2011) Abnormal plasticity in dystonia: disruption of synaptic homeostasis. *Neurobiol. Dis.* **42**, 162–170.

Raichle, M.E. and Snyder, A.Z. (2007) A default mode of brain function: a brief history of an evolving idea. *NeuroImage* **37**, 1083–1090.

Ramel, W., Goldin, P.R., Carmona, P.E. and McQuaid, J.R. (2004) The effects of mindfulness meditation on cognitive processes and affect in patients with past depression. *Cognitive. Ther. Res.* **28**, 433–455.

Raz, A. and Buhle, J. (2006) Typologies of attentional networks. *Nat. Rev. Neurosci.* **7**, 367–379.

Rojas Vega, S., Abel, T., Lindschulten, R., Hollmann, W., Bloch, W. and Strüder, H.K. (2008) Impact of exercise on neuroplasticity-related proteins in spinal cord injured humans. *Neuroscience* **153**, 1064–1070.

Sagula, D. and Rice, K.G. (2004) The effectiveness of mindfulness training on the grieving process and emotional well-being of chronic pain patients. *J. Clin. Psychol. Med. Settings* **11**, 333–342.

Salzberg, S. (1995) *Lovingkindness: The Revolutionary Art of Happiness*, 1st Ed. Shambhala, Boston, MA.

Sanes, J.R. and Lichtman, J.W. (1999) Can molecules explain long-term potentiation? *Nat. Neurosci.* **2**, 597.

Tang, Y-Y., Ma, Y., Wang, J., Fan, Y., Feng, S., Lu, Q., Yu, Q., Sui, D., Rothbart, M.K., Fan, M. and Posner, M.I. (2007) Short-term meditation training improves attention and self-regulation. *Proc. Natl. Acad. Sci. USA* **104**, 17152–17156.

Travis, F., Haaga, D., Hagelin, J., Tanner, M., Arenander, A., Nidich, S., Gaylord-King, C., Grosswald, S., Rainforth, M. and Schneider, R. (2010) A self-referential default brain state: patterns of coherence, power, and eLORETA sources during eyes-closed rest and transcendental meditation practice. *Cogn. Process* **11**, 21–30.

Vestergaard-Poulsen, P., van Beek, M., Skewes, J., Bjarkam, C.R., Stubberup, M., Bertelsen, J. and Roepstorff, A. (2009) Long-term meditation is associated with increased gray matter density in the brain stem. *Neuroreport* **20**, 170–174.

Wang, K., Fan, J., Dong, Y., Wang, C.-Q., Lee, T.M.C. and Posner, M.I. (2005) Selective impairment of attentional networks of orienting and executive control in schizophrenia. *Schizophr. Res.* **78**, 235–241.

Williams, A.-L., Selwyn, P.A., Liberti, L., Molde, S., Njike, V.Y., McCorkle, R., Zelterman, D. and Katz, D.L. (2005) A randomized controlled trial of meditation and massage effects on quality of life in people with late-stage disease: a pilot study. *J. Palliat. Med.* **8**, 939–952.

Zeidan, F., Gordon, N.S., Merchant, J. and Goolkasian, P. (2010) The effects of brief mindfulness meditation training on experimentally induced pain. *J. Pain* **11**, 199–209.

Zgierska, A., Rabago, D., Zuelsdorff, M., Coe, C., Miller, M. and Fleming, M. (2008) Mindfulness meditation for alcohol relapse prevention: a feasibility pilot study. *J. Addict. Med.* **2**, 165–173.

Zylowska, L., Ackerman, D.L., Yang, M.H., Futrell, J.L., Horton, N.I., Hale, T.S., Pataki, C. and Smalley, S.L. (2008) Mindfulness meditation training in adults and adolescents with ADHD: a feasibility study. *J. Atten. Disord.* **11**, 737–746.

Chapter 11

Shaolin Mind-Body Exercise as a Neuropsychological Intervention

Agnes Suiyin Chan and Sophia Laiman Sze

Abstract

Mind-body exercise, a form of physical exercise originating in the East with increasing popularity in the West, has a unique characteristic that requires conscious control of each body movement and concurrently maintaining a peaceful and relaxed state of mind during practice. With the ultimate goal of training both the body and the mind, there have been empirical findings supporting the positive effects of mind-body exercises on improving physical health condition (e.g., pulmonary function) as well as cognitive functions (e.g., learning and memory). This chapter will introduce a form of Chinese *Chan*-based mind-body exercise, namely *Shaolin* mind-body exercise or *Chanwu*, which was developed upon the traditional *Shaolin* Healing Approach. A brief description on some movements of *Shaolin* mind-body exercise will also be provided. Treatment outcomes based on both clinical observations and cumulative empirical evidence are so far encouraging. Specifically, intervention with the component of *Shaolin* mind-body exercise has been found to be able to foster a relaxed and attentive mind state of normal adults, significantly improve depressive mood and enhance bowel function and neurophysiological activity of both community-dwelling adults and patients with major depressive disorder. Some clinical cases with severe cognitive impairment have also been assessed to show significant enhancement in their attention, memory, language and executive functions. These positive findings have suggested potential clinical applicability of the *Shaolin* mind-body exercise as a possible neuropsychological intervention for improving cognitive function and psychological status of patients with various brain disorders or psychiatric illnesses.

Keywords: Mind-Body exercise; Physical Health; Mood; Cognitive Function; Brain Disorder.

11.1 Exercises Improve the Cognitive Functions

There have been many studies, both on animals and humans, that point to the positive effect of exercises on cognitive functions. Some animal studies have examined the effect of exercise on the brain-derived neurotrophic factor (BDNF) with positive findings reported (Gomez-Pinilla *et al.*, 2011; Vaynman *et al.*, 2004), and have reported that exercise enhanced their memory as indicated by their improved performance on the Morris water maze (Vaynman *et al.*, 2004). Some studies investigating the effect of exercise on hippocampus (Brown *et al.*, 2003; Van Praag *et al.*, 1999; Trejo *et al.*, 2001; Eadie *et al.*, 2005) have consistently reported increasing cell proliferation and cell survival in the dentate gyrus of the hippocampus.

Human studies consistently showed positive effects of exercises on improving cognitive function across the life-span. A meta-analysis reported a positive relationship between physical activity, and cognitive function and academic performance in children (Sibley and Etnier, 2003). A study explored the effect of a half-year home-based exercise program, in which the children were requested to do some spinning, bouncing, walking and throwing at home. After six months, students who have reading difficulty demonstrated improved reading accuracy, phonemic skill, working memory and attention (Reynolds and Nicolson, 2007). In addition, college students performed better in tasks testing reaction time and vocabulary learning after running (Hillman *et al.*, 2003; Winter *et al.*, 2007).

In aging populations, studies showed that regular exercise is a protective factor against cognitive decline, such as executive planning and working memory (Kramer *et al.*, 1999; Barnes *et al.*, 2003; Colcombe and Kramer, 2003). A three-month exercise intervention improved the depressive symptoms in individuals with Alzheimer's disease (Teri *et al.*, 2003). In a magnetic resonance imaging (MRI) study on the brain volume of a group of 60–79 years old adults, the results showed that those who participated in aerobic exercise training, as compared to the control group, demonstrated increased brain volume in the frontal lobe regions (Colcombe *et al.*, 2006). In another study, older adults were randomly assigned into either aerobic exercise group or wait-list group. After ten weeks of intervention, individuals participated in the aerobic training program showed significant improvement in a dual auditory and visual discrimination tasks (Hawkins *et al.*, 1992).

Interesting enough, the benefit of exercise on cognitive function is not correlated with the cardiovascular fitness, that is, higher level of fitness does not necessary lead to larger cognitive improvement (Etnier *et al*, 2006). On the other hand, exercise program consisting of balancing, timing and co-ordination showed significant benefit to the reading abilities of children with dyslexia (Reynolds and Nicolson, 2007). This finding suggests that the benefit of exercise is not necessarily restricted to cardiovascular exercise or the intensity of practice.

Mind-body (MB) exercise is a form of physical exercise long used in the East and now increasingly popular in the West. A unique characteristic of MB exercises is that they emphasize the conscious control of each body movement. To pay attention to each movement, the exercises typically involve slow motion. Moreover, those who perform it are requested to maintain a peaceful and relaxed state of mind. Although the movement of MB exercises in general is relatively slow, some are classified as moderate-intensity exercise with similar physiological benefits as cardiovascular exercises such as improving pulmonary function (Hong *et al.*, 2000; Lai *et al.,* 1995) and reduced blood pressure (Thornton *et al.*, 2004; Tsai *et al.*, 2003). A study compared the memory function of older adults who regularly practiced mind-body (MB) exercise or cardiovascular (CV) exercises, and the results showed that older adults practicing MB or CV exercises demonstrated a similar level of memory function, and their learning and memory was better than those who did not exercise regularly (Chan *et al.*, 2005).

11.2 The *Shaolin* Mind-Body Exercise

In the past several years, our research team has devoted to study the effect of the *Shaolin* mind-body exercise as a possible neuropsychological intervention for improving the cognitive function and/or psychological status of patients with brain disorders or psychiatric disorders.

The *Shaolin* mind-body exercise is a special form of Martial Arts that have been developed within the *Shaolin* Temple, and is also called *Chanwu* (禪武). The purpose of *Chanwu* is to train the mind and the heart but not the muscle; thus, it focuses on the internal practice rather than training the muscles and the limbs. The internal practice is the practice of the mind in which the mind needs to be always calm and quiet. When the mind is calm, the *Qi* is strong, and strong *Qi* is internal energy. Otherwise, the *Qi* is disrupted and there is lack of internal energy. It should be noted that the *Shaolin* Temple used to be divided into different branches: North, East, South, and West. The mind-body exercises that we have studied were passed down from the South branch. This form of mind-body exercise that we studied, named *Nei Yang Gong* (內養功), consists of *Dan Tian* Breathing Exercises, Tranquil Stand, Shoulder Relaxation, and Nasal Bridge Massage. The *Dan Tian* Breathing Exercises have both Passive *Dan Tian* Breathing and Active *Dan Tian* Breathing. Passive *Dan Tian* Breathing can be practiced either at sitting or standing posture. Put one or both hands gently on the abdomen below the navel, and close both eyes gently. Passively observe the abdomen when breathing in, and observe the nose when breathing out. Active *Dan Tian* Breathing is similar to Passive *Dan Tian* Breathing except when breathing out, contract the anus and the abdomen gently, close the mouth, and open the eyes. When breathing in, close the eyes and relax the whole body. To practice Tranquil Stand, one stands squarely on both feet to about the shoulders' width and raises the hands gently in front of the chest, like a standing monkey. The eyes and mouth close slightly, push the tongue to the roof of the oral cavity gently, and stand quietly for five to thirty minutes. The "action *gong*" includes the Shoulder Relaxation and Nasal Bridge Massage. Shoulder Relaxation is performed by placing both hands in the middle of the shoulders and the neck, and then using the shoulders to lead the arms to make a circular motion. When one is familiar with this, one can also bend the lower back a little forward and lift the heels. The Nasal Bridge Massage is performed by gently massaging the left and the right sides of the nose bridge with the two index fingers.

For the past years, our research team has conducted studies to examine the effect of this *Shaolin* Kung Fu on improving the cognitive and psychological health of community dwelling adults (Chan *et al.*, 2011b), patients with depression (Chan *et al.*, 2012a; 2012b), children with autism (Chan *et al.*, 2008, 2011c, 2013), and patients with various forms of brain disorders (Chan *et al.*, 2009). However, it should be noted that according to the *Shaolin* Healing Approach, the effect of *Chanwu* will be enhanced with the special diet modification that aims to reduce the internal heat and *Qi* blockage. The diet modification recommends reducing intake of meat, fish and egg. Some of the vegetables are also suggested to avoid as they are considered "*hun cai*", including spring onion, Chinese chives and garlic. In addition, ginger, mustard and hot spices should be avoided. According to the *Shaolin* medicine, meat, hot and spicy foods have high protein, high fat, and high energy content that will over stimulate the *Qi* and blood circulation. If they are not properly digested, they will stay inside the body and cause inflammation of the body and affect the blood and *Qi* circulation. The blockage of blood and *Qi* circulation and the inflammation inside the body will significantly affect the mental and physical condition adversely. Thus, diet modification is a significant condition for the *Shaolin* mind-body exercises to have positive effect on improving mental and physical health.

In one of the studies (Chan *et al.*, 2011a), we aimed to investigate the neuroelectrophysiological response of the *Shaolin Dan Tian* Breathing (DTB) technique, which consists of the Passive and Active subtypes. It was hypothesized that this breathing exercise, which is a form of *Nei Yang Gong*, would induce both relaxed and attentive states of mind. The rationale for examining this neurophysiological phenomenon was that some empirical studies have suggested that enhancing both a relaxed and an attentive mind state is crucial for achieving higher cognitive performance, such as enhanced attention and concentration, faster reaction time, better decision making ability and increased creativity, and thereby improving work efficiency and productivity. Thus, if the *Shaolin Dan Tian* Breathing can lead to a relaxed and attentive state of mind, it will provide some neuro-based explanation for its positive effect on enhancing cognitive function and psychological status in adults and children.

In this study, forty-four adults were randomly assigned to receive either training on the *Shaolin* DTB (experimental group) or progressive muscle relaxation for one month. Eyes-closed resting EEG data before and immediately after each type of breathing were obtained individually at baseline and after one-month training. At baseline, the EEG changes after the *Shaolin* DTB between both groups were comparable. After one-month training, participants in the experimental, but not the control, group showed enhanced temporal alpha asymmetry (an index of relaxation and positive mood) after performing the Passive DTB for five minutes, and enhanced intra- and inter-hemispheric theta coherence (an index of attention and alertness) after performing the Active DTB (Fig. 1). The results showed that participants in the experimental but not the control group showed enhanced temporal alpha asymmetry and theta coherence levels after the one-month practice, with a mean practicing time of 15 minutes per day. These results suggested that practicing the *Shaolin* DTB facilitated the attainment of the co-existing states of relaxed and attentive mind, which made this breathing technique uniquely different from other more well-known breathing techniques. Specifically, the majority of the electrophysiological studies on meditative breathing reported either elevated anterior alpha asymmetry (Davidson *et al.*, 2003; Barnhofer *et al.*, 2007) or theta coherence (Aftanas and Golocheikine, 2001; 2003), but rarely both (Takahashi *et al.*, 2005). The *Shaolin* DTB technique, on the other hand, seemed to be able to enhance both temporal alpha asymmetry and theta coherence, suggesting that this technique may be useful to induce a relaxed and attentive mind state.

The principle for the development of the *Shaolin* DTB was based upon Chinese martial arts and *Qigong* that cannot be fully explicable using western concepts. Specifically, the *Shaolin* DTB consists of two forms, Passive and Active, that need to be practiced together alternately, for instance, practicing five times Passive DTB and once Active DTB, or ten times Passive DTB and thrice Active DTB (the frequency depends on the individual's feeling). The rationale for practicing the DTB this way was to enhance the blood and *Qi* circulation more effectively. Thus, the *Shaolin* DTB is not simply a relaxation exercise but also a form of *Qigong*. Results from the present study showed that practicing the DTB not only induced a relaxed (i.e., temporal alpha asymmetry) but also an attentive (i.e., theta coherence) state of mind, which has provided some pilot data supporting the rationale that the *Shaolin* DTB is more than a relaxation exercise.

In another study (Chan *et al.*, 2011b) that evaluated the effectiveness of the *Shaolin* Healing approach for improving the depressive mood of an adult community sample, forty adult volunteers with various degrees of depressive mood were randomly assigned to the experimental group (*Dejian* Mind-Body Intervention, DMBI) in which learning the *Shaolin Chanwu* is one of the major component, and the control group receiving the Cognitive-Behavioral Therapy (CBT). For each group, a total of four 90-minute weekly sessions were conducted. The individuals were measured at pre- and post-treatment with various psychological and health assessments. Treatment-related changes were measured using the Beck Depression Inventory (BDI-II), an electroencephalographic indicator of positive affect (i.e., prefrontal activation asymmetry), and self-report ratings on physical health. Results indicated that both the DMBI and the CBT group demonstrated significant reduction in depressive mood. However, among individuals with moderate to severe depressive mood at baseline, only those in the DMBI but not the CBT group showed significant reduction in depressive mood (Fig. 2). Besides, only participants of the DMBI but not the CBT group showed a significant leftward shift of the frontal asymmetry index after treatment, which signifies a significant increase in positive affect/mood. In addition, participants of the DMBI reported significant treatment-related improvement in their bowel condition, while no such improvement was reported among participants of the CBT. Consistent with the self-reports, the quantified interview data revealed that out of the three parameters of bowel condition, significant improvements were found on two (i.e., amount of time for emptying the bowel, and the feeling of incomplete emptying of the bowel after defecation) in the DMBI group, while no improvement was found in the CBT group (Fig. 3). These results provided initial empirical evidence suggesting that the DMBI has positive effects on both the mind (i.e., depressive mood) and the body (i.e., bowel condition). It should be noted that the improvement of bowel function has not yet been reported as a treatment outcome for most psychological therapies; thus the mind-body intervention approach seems to have an additional therapeutic effect besides psychological intervention. While most psychological therapies for depressive mood normally take several months to show treatment effect, the present findings provided initial data suggesting that the *Dejian* Mind-Body Intervention was effective in improving depressive mood of community adults after one month of training. In a follow-up study (Chan *et al.*, 2012), we examined the effects of the *Shaolin Chanwu* on patients with clinical depression who were receiving medical treatment. Seventy-five participants diagnosed with major depressive disorder were randomly assigned to receive either ten-session CBT or DMBI, or placed on a waitlist. Both the CBT and DMBI groups demonstrated significantly reduced overall depressive syndrome after intervention. Furthermore, the DMBI group, but not the CBT or waitlist groups, demonstrated significant reduction in intake of anti-depressants (Fig. 4), and significant improvement in specific depression-related symptoms including difficulty in concentration, and problems in gastrointestinal health and overall sleep quality. In sum, the *Shaolin Chanwu* seems to have a positive effect in community sample as well as in clinical population for improving the mental health, cognitive function and physical health.

Besides, we have applied the *Chanwu* and the *Shaolin* Healing Approach — *Chanwuyi* in our rehabilitation center for the past years, and the clinical outcomes on case studies so far are encouraging. There was a 22-year-old chronic epileptic male, who had the illness onset at age two, suffering from severe cognitive impairments as a result of a serious seizure two years ago when time to receive the intervention in our center (Chan *et al.*, 2009). The patient has undergone the *Shaolin* Medical Healing process in which *Chanwu* is one of the major components. Through a four-month treatment, the patient showed significant improvements in language, memory, attention, behavioral initiation, emotional control, social functioning, and overall quality of life. In addition, there was a positive effect on his brain electrophysiological activities, as indicated by his suppressed delta power (slow wave) and enhanced alpha power (fast wave), and his elevated cordance value (an index associated with cerebral perfusion) in the left frontal and temporal regions. Such neural activity alteration was in line with his observed cognitive improvement. Thus, these results provide evidence to support the therapeutic effect of the *Shaolin* Healing approach and its potential clinical application on treating chronic neurological patients. Similarly, there is another case of a teenage girl, TK, diagnosed with Asperger's disorder (Chan *et al.*, 2008). She has been instructed to practice the *Shaolin* mind-body exercise as a way to improve her self-control ability. Instant intervention effect on TK was noted with significant reduction in temper tantrums and repetitive behaviors, and faster self-calming process after the first week of intervention. The effect was sustainable throughout the three-month intervention period. Additional positive changes in problem-solving and psychosocial functioning were also observed. Similar effects were observed on a nine-year-old boy with low-functioning autism, KY (Chan *et al.*, 2011c). After a one month intervention with the *Shaolin* Healing method, the child's inhibitory control, cognitive flexibility, and memory functioning have significantly improved from "severely-to-moderately impaired" to "within-normal" range. This improvement was not observed from previous a 12-month conventional cognitive intervention. Furthermore, KY showed increased cordance gradually extending from the anterior to the posterior brain region, suggesting possible neural mechanism underlying his cognitive improvement. These findings have implicated potential applicability of the *Shaolin* Healing Approach and the *Shaolin* mind-body exercise as a rehabilitation program for patients with cognitive impairment.

References

Aftanas, L.I. and Golocheikine, S.A. (2001) Human anterior and frontal midline theta and lower alpha reflect emotionally positive state and internalized attention: high-resolution EEG investigation of meditation. *Neurosci. Lett.* **310**, 57–60.

Aftanas, L.I. and Golocheikine, S.A. (2003) Changes in cortical activity in altered states of consciousness: the study of meditation by high-resolution EEG. *Hum. Physiol.* **29**, 143–151.

Barnes, D.E., Yaffe, K., Satariano, W.A. and Tager, I.B. (2003) A longitudinal study of cardiorespiratory fitness and cognitive function in healthy older adults. *J. Am. Geriatr. Soc.* **51**, 459–465.

Barnhofer, T., Duggan, D., Crane, C., Hepburn, S., Fennell, M.J.V. and Williams, J.M.G. (2007) Effects of meditation on frontal and asymmetry in previously suicidal individuals. *Neuroreport* **18**, 709–712.

Brown, J., Cooper-Kuhn, C.M., Kempermann, G., Van Praag, H., Winkler, J., Gage, F.H. and Kuhn, H.G. (2003). Enriched environment and physical activity stimulate hippocampal but not olfactory bulb neurogenesis. *Eur. J. Neurosci.* **17**, 2042–2046.

Chan, A.S., Ho, Y.C., Cheung, M.C., Albert, M.S. Chiu, H.F. and Lam, L.C. (2005) Association between mind-body and cardiovascular exercises and memory in older adults. *J. Am. Geriatr. Soc.* **53**, 1754–1760.

Chan, A.S., Sze, S.L. and Shi, D. (2008) Traditional Chinese mind-body exercises improve self control ability of an adolescent with Asperger's disorder. *J. Psychol. Chin. Soc.* **9**, 225–239.

Chan, A.S., Sze, S.L., Cheung, M.C., Lam, J.M.K. and Shi, D. (2009) *Dejian* mind-body intervention improves the functioning of a patient with chronic epilepsy: a case report. *Cases J.* DOI:10.1186/1757-1626-2-9080.

Chan, A.S., Cheung, M.C., Sze, S.L., Leung, W.W. and Shi, D. (2011a) *Shaolin Dan Tian* breathing fosters relaxed and attentive mind: a randomized controlled neuroelectrophysiological study. *Evid. Based Complement. Altern. Med.* DOI:10.1155/2011/180704.

Chan, A.S., Cheung, M.C., Tsui, W.J., Sze, S.L. and Shi, D. (2011b) *Dejian* mind-body intervention on depressive mood of community-dwelling adults: a randomized controlled trial. *Evid. Based Complement. Altern. Med.* DOI:10.1093/ecam/nep043.

Chan, A.S., Sze S.L., Cheung, M.C., Han, Y.M.Y., Leung, W.W.M. and Shi, D. (2011c) *Dejian* mind-body intervention improves the cognitive functions of a child with autism. *Evid. Based Complement. Altern. Med.* DOI:10.1155/2011/549254.

Chan, A.S., Wong, Q.Y., Sze, S.L., Kwong, P.P.K., Han, Y.M.Y. and Cheung, M.C. (2012a) A Chinese *Chan*-based mind-body intervention for patients with depression. *J. Affect. Disorders* **142**, 283–289.

Chan, A.S., Wong, Q.Y., Sze, S.L., Kwong, P.P.K., Han, Y.M.Y. and Cheung, M.C. (2012b) A Chinese *Chan*-based mind-body intervention improves sleep on patients with depression: a randomized controlled trial. *Scientific World J.* DOI:10.1100/2012/235206

Chan, A.S., Sze, S.L., Siu, N.Y. and Cheung, M.C. (2013) A Chinese mind-body exercise improves self-control of children with autism: a randomized controlled trial (under review).

Colcombe, S. and Kramer, A.F. (2003) Fitness effects on the cognitive function of older adults: a meta-analytic study. *Psychol. Sci.* **14**, 125–130.

Colcombe, S.J., Erickson, K.I., Scalf, P.E., Kim, J.S., Prakash, R., McAuley, E., Elavsky, S., Marquez, D.X., Hu, L. and Kramer, A.F. (2006) Aerobic exercise training increases brain volume in aging humans. *J. Gerontol.* **61A**, 1166–1170.

Davidson, R.J., Kabat-Zinn, J., Schumacher, J., Rosenkranz, M., Muller, D., Santorelli, S.F., Urbanowski, F., Harrington, A., Bonus, K. and Sheridan, J.F. (2003) Alterations in brain and immune function produced by mindfulness meditation. *Psychosom. Med.* **65**, 564–570.

Eadie, B.D., Redilla, V.A. and Christie, B.R. (2005) Voluntary exercise alters the cytoarchitecture of the adult dentate gyrus by increasing cellular proliferation, dendritic complexity, and spine density. *J. Comp. Neurol.* **486**, 39–47.

Etnier, J.L., Nowell, P.M., Landers, D.M. and Sibley, B.A. (2006) A meta-regression to examine the relationship between aerobic fitness and cognitive performance. *Brain Res Rev.* **52**, 119–130.

Gomez-Pinilla, F., Zhuang, Y., Feng, J., Ying, Z. and Fan, G. (2011) Exercise impacts brain-derived neurotrophic factor plasticity by engaging mechanisms of epigenetic regulation. *Eur. J. Neurosci.* **33**, 383–390.

Hawkins, H.L., Kramer, A.F. and Capaldi, D. (1992) Aging, exercise and attention. *Psychol. Aging* **7**: 643–653.

Hillman, C.H., Snook, E.M. and Jerome, G.J. (2003) Acute cardiovascular exercise and executive control function. *Int. J. Psychophysiol.* **48**, 307–314.

Hong, Y, Li, J.X. and Robinson, P.D. (2000) Effects of long-term Tai Chi exercise on balance, flexibility, and cardiovascular response in the elderly. *Br. J. Sports Med.* **34**, 29–34.

Kramer, A.F., Hahn, S., Cohen, N.J., Banich, M.T., McAuley, E., Harrison, C.R., Chason, J., Vakil, E., Bardell, L., Boileau, R.A. and Colcombe, A. (1999) Ageing, fitness and neurocognitive function. *Nature* **400**, 418–419.

Lai, J.S., Lan, C., Wong, M.K. and Teng, S.H. (1995) Two-year trends in cardiorespiratory function among older Tai Chi Chuan practitioners and sedentary subjects. *J. Am. Geriatr. Soc.* **43**, 1222–1227.

Reynolds, D. and Nicolson, R.I. (2007) Follow-up of an exercise-based treatment for children with reading difficulties. *Dyslexia* **13**, 78–96.

Sibley, B.A. and Etnier, J.L. (2003) The relationship between physical activity and cognition in children: a meta-analysis. *Pediatr. Exerc. Sci.* **15**, 243–256.

Takahashi, T., Murata, T., Hamada, T., Omori, M., Kosaka, H., Kikuchi, M., Yoshida, H. and Wada, Y. (2005) Changes in EEG and autonomic nervous activity during meditation and their association with personality traits. *Int. J. Psychophysiol.* **55**, 199–207.

Teri, L., Gibbons, L.E., McCurry, S.M., Logsdon, R.G., Buchner, D.M., Barlow, W.E., Kukull, W.A., LaCroix, A.X., McCormick, W. and Larson, E.B. (2003) Exercise plus behavioural management in patients with Alzheimer's disease: a randomized controlled trail. *J. Am. Med. Assoc.* **290**, 2015–2022.

Thornton, E.W., Sykes, K.S. and Tang, W.K. (2004) Health benefits of Tai Chi exercise: improved balance and blood pressure in middle-aged women. *Health Promot. Int.* **19**, 22–38.

Trejo, J.L., Carro, E. and Torres-Aleman, I. (2001) Circulating insulin-like growth factor mediates exercise-induced increases in the number of new neurons in the adult hippocampus. *J. Neurosci.* **21**, 1628–1634.

Tsai, J.C., Wang, W.H., Chan, P., Lin, L.J., Wang, C.H., Tomlinson, B., Hsieh, M.H., Yang, H.Y. and Liu, J.C. (2003) The beneficial effects of Tai Chi Chuan on blood pressure and lipid profile and anxiety status in a randomized controlled trail. *J. Altern. Complement. Med.* **9**, 747–754.

Van Praag, H., Kempermann, G. and Gage, F.H. (1999) Running increases cell proliferation and neurogensis in the adult mouse dentate gyrus. *Nat. Neurosci.* **2**, 266–270.

Vaynman, S., Ying, Z. and Gomez-Pinilla, F. (2004) Hippocampal BDNF mediates the efficacy of exercise on synaptic plasticity and cognition. *Eur. J. Neurosci.* **20**, 2580–2590.

Winter, B., Breitenstein, C., Mooren, F.C., Voelker, K., Fobker, M., Lechtermann, A., Krueger, K., Fromme, A., Korsukewitz, C., Floel, A. and Knecht, S. (2007) High impact running improves learning. *Neurobiol. Learn. Mem.* **87**, 597–609.

Chapter 12

Near-Infrared (NIR) Spectroscopy as a Tool for Quality Control of Traditional Chinese Herbal Medicines

Lukas Bittner, Stefan Schönbichler and Christian Huck

Abstract

Traditional Chinese Medicine (TCM) is increasing in popularity all over the world. However, due to the high demand for TCM products, quality control becomes a challenge as many formulations have a complicated composition. Moreover, in addition to quantitative control of ingredients, the geographic origin and the species must be identified. Analytical techniques employed so far, including mass spectroscopy, NMR spectroscopy and separation techniques, are all destructive, expensive and time-consuming, and therefore they are not really suitable for high-throughput quality control. For this purpose, near-infrared (NIR) offers novel highly and effective possibilities for a very fast, non-invasive and simultaneous investigation of a manifold of different questions. The present chapter aims to point out the efficiency of modern NIR methodology in addressing the above-mentioned problems through several well-selected examples. Thus, this contribution should help to convince the implementation of such an analytical method in quality control at different stages of the production process.

Keywords: Near-Infrared Spectroscopy; Quality Control; Non-Invasive; Fast Analysis; Authentication; Geographical Identification; Quantitation; Simultaneous Measurement.

12.1 Introduction

Traditional Chinese medicine (TCM), with its more than 5000 years old history of clinical application, is of increasing importance also outside of China, especially in Europe and North America. In China the use of traditional herbal medicinal products constitute between 30% and 50% of the total consumption of medicines, which has a sales value of USD14 billion in 2005. In Europe the total sales of herbal medicines equals USD5 billion in 2003 with Germany and France counting 60% of this value, and the market was growing significantly over the last years (De Smet, 2005).

Figure 12.1(a) shows the percentage of persons in developed countries who have used complementary and alternative medicine at least once. Whilst the majority of the countries have listed between one and ten herbal medicines on their national essential drug lists, China is the extreme with

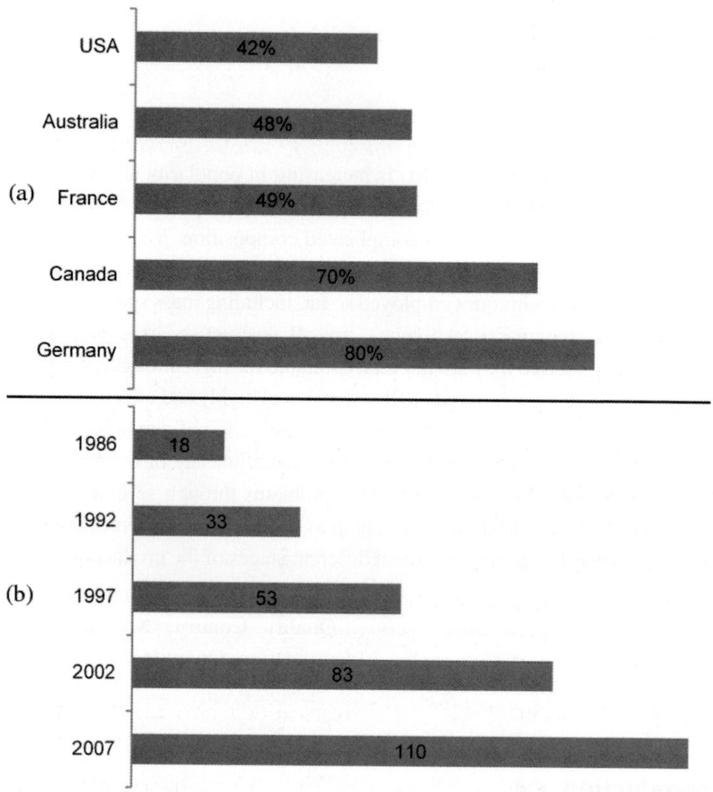

Figure 12.1. (a) Populations in developed countries who have used complementary and alternative medicine at least once. (b) WHO member states having regulations or laws governing herbal medicines.

Source: Robinson and Zhang (2011).

1242 essential herbal medicines and more than 9000 herbal medicines in its pharmacopeia. An increasing number of countries have regulations or laws governing herbal medicines as can be seen in Fig. 12.1(b) (Robinson and Zhang, 2011).

To ensure quality in TCM it is necessary to have analytical methods for authentication of plant material and origin, quantitative and qualitative analysis of its compounds and identification of different parts of the plants. Methods such as liquid chromatography (LC), capillary electrophoresis (CE) or mass spectrometry (MS) are well established and highly efficient analytical tools, but have also disadvantages such as expensive instrumentation, the necessity of special trained operators or high time consumption. Near-infrared (NIR) spectroscopy is an alternative and with its well-known advantages a low-cost and high-throughput analytical tool (Guo *et al.*, 2011).

In the following an overview of the latest research of NIR spectroscopy in TCM is given.

12.2 Applications

NIR spectroscopy has been deployed for qualitative and quantitative analysis of single compounds in plant materials for a long time (Huck *et al.*, 1999; 2006), and is used throughout the phyto-pharmaceutical production process from raw material to production and extraction processes until the final medicinal formulation (Guo *et al.*, 2011).

Xiang *et al.* (2002) described a method to use NIR spectroscopy in combination with artificial neural networks (ANN) to discriminate between official (listed in the Chinese pharmacopeia) and unofficial medicinal *rhubarb*. A neural network with eight input nodes, a 0.5 learning rate and a momentum of 0.3 can achieve a prediction accuracy of 96.8% for the test set. Tang and coworkers (2004) did similar experiments getting a prediction accuracy of 98%. Zhao *et al.* (2008) showed that using Fisher classification wavelet packet entropy (WPE) lead to lower error rates than principal component analysis (PCA) for the classification of medicinal *rhubarbs*. Figure 12.2 shows how wild and cultivated *radix scutellariae* can be distinguished deploying NIR spectroscopy in combination with PCA. Chan *et al.* (2007) differentiated two species of *cortex phellodendri*

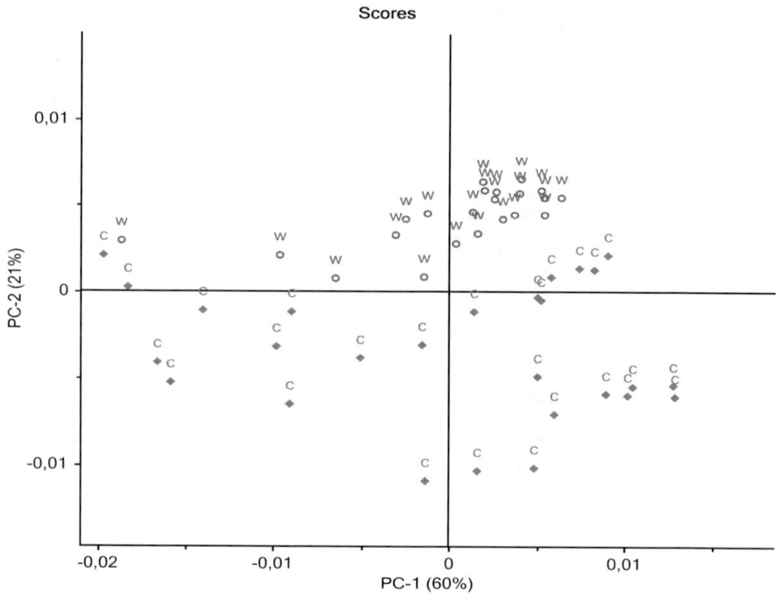

Figure 12.2. Principal components score plot of wild and cultivated Radix scutellariae samples (unpublished results).

and predicted quantitatively berberine and total alkaloid content applying parital least square regression (PLSR). A number of researches developed NIR spectroscopic methods to confirm the geographic origin of raw plant material ("geoherbs"). Deriving from traditional beliefs, the geographical origin of medicinal herbs plays a decisive role as a sales argument. Lai and coworkers (2011) developed a method to determine the geographical origin of *rhizoma corydalis* comparing the performances of least-squares support vector machines (LS-SVM), radial basis function ANN (RBF-ANN), partial least square discriminant analysis (PLS-DA) and K-nearest neighbors (KNN) methods. LS-SVM performed best classifying over 95% of the samples correctly. Woo and coworkers (2002) distinguished Chinese from Korean *ginseng* by deploying soft independent modeling of class analogy (SIMCA). Han *et al.*, (2009) compared different data analysis methods to confirm the geographic origin of *radix pseudostellariae* with the SVM model showing the best performance. Chen and coworkers (2008) applied PCA, PLS-DA and discriminant analysis (DA) to discriminate *ganoderma lucidum* according to its cultivation area in three

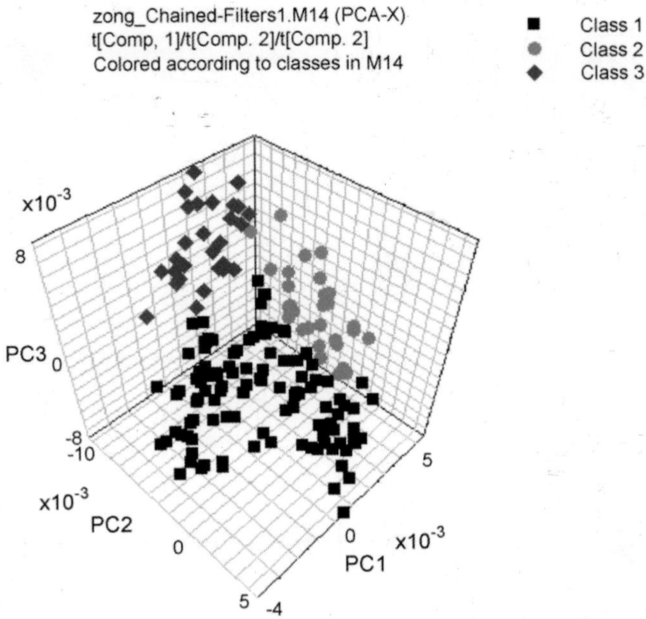

Figure 12.3. Three-dimensional scoreplot (PC1, PC2, PC3) to discriminate between Gandoderma ludicum from Shandong (Class 1), Anhui (Class 2) and Zhejiang (Class 3). Reproduced with permission from Chen *et al.* (2008).

different provinces of China. Figure 12.3 shows a three-dimensional score plot separating *ganoderma lucidum* from Shandon, Anhui and Zhejiang provinces. Licorice, the root of *glycyrrhiza uralensis Fisch*, is widely used a medicinal herb as well as a food additive due to its sweet taste originating from glyzirrhizin, a glycoside in the combines potassium and sodium salt of glycyrrhizic acid (GA). Wang *et al.*, (2007) successfully developed a system to cluster licorice based on geographic areas, growing conditions and plant parts as well as a partial least square regression (PLSR) model to predict the GA content. Lu and coworkers (2008) applied temperature-induced two-dimensional NIR correlation spectroscopy to determine the geographic origin of *fructus lycii*. Figure 12.4 displays the 2D correlation asynchronous spectra of *fructus lycii* in a wavenumber range from 4950 cm^{-1} to 5700 cm^{-1} from four different regions. Wu *et al.*, (2010) studied the differences between epidermis, phloem and xylem of *radix ginseng*. Lau and coworkers (2009) developed a system to classify the

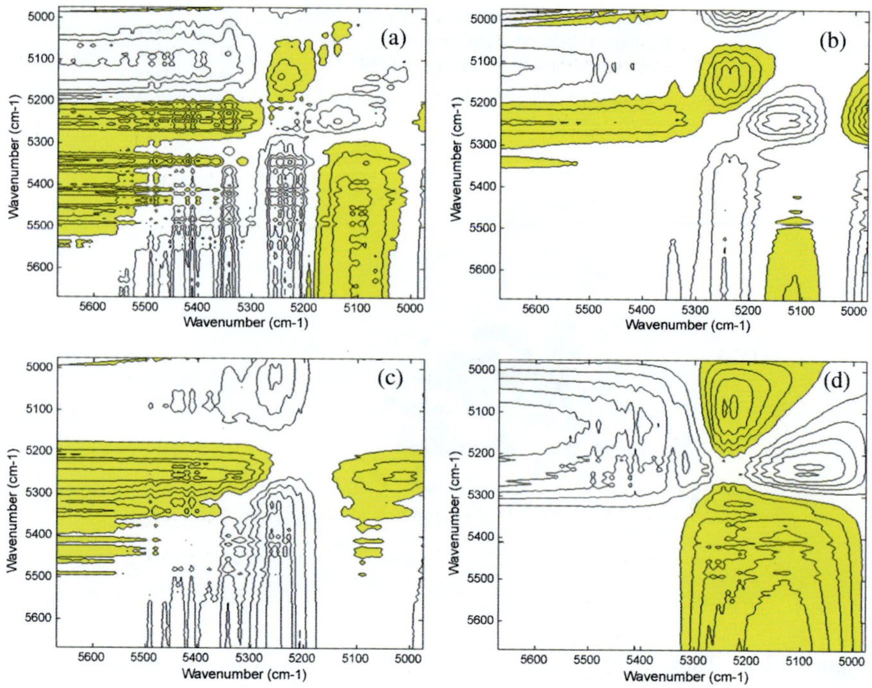

Figure 12.4. 2D correlation NIR asynchronous spectra of Fructus Lycii samples. (a) Ningxia, (b) Inner Mongolia, (c) Hebei, and (d) Sinkiang. Yellow areas represent negative crosspeaks. Reproduced with permission from Lu *et al.* (2008).

species of *radix puerariae* and simultaneously predict quantitatively the contents of puerarin, daidzin and total isoflavonoids.

Li *et al.* (2010) created calibration models to predict chlorogenic acid, caffeic acid, luteoloside, baicalin, ursodesoxycholic acid (UDCA) and chenodeoxycholic acid (CDCA) quantitatively in *Tanreqing* injection intermediates. *Tanreqing* injection is a patented drug widely used in China consisting of extracts of five different medicinal herbs used for treatment of various diseases. Fu and coworkers (2009) used NIR spectroscopy to identify *Liuwei Dihuang* Pills from different manufacturers deploying moving window partial least squares discriminant analysis (MWPLSDA). Nanlin *et al.* (2003) determined the mannitol content in fermented *cordyceps sinensis* powder using ANN. Wu *et al.* (2008) used NIRS and mid-infrared spectroscopy (MIR) in combination with PLSR for quality assessment of *Honghua* oil, a preparation consisting of various etheric oils, developing prediction models for the three marker components α-pinene, methyl salycilate and eugenol. Rosa and coworkers (2008) applied NIRS as a process analytical technology (PAT) tool for qualitative quality control of *ginkgo biloba* extract.

12.3 Perspective

In 2005 NIR spectroscopy was included in the Chinese pharmacopeia as an official method for quality control of TCM (Guo *et al.*, 2011). In recent publications NIR spectroscopy for TCM is of growing importance with Jiang *et al.*, (2010) assigning it one chapter in his review about quality control in TCM. With its advantages of on- and in-line measurements, high throughput and relative low costs, NIR spectroscopy offers a huge potential for applications in the phyto-pharmaceutical industry, especially regarding the adoption of PAT.

Another aspect which has to be considered is product safety, especially possible contaminations in herbal products such as pesticides, microbial contaminants, heavy metals or chemical toxins (Liang *et al.*, 2004).

As some traditional Chinese medicinal formulations are prepared from plant juices there is the possibility that the aquaphotomics approach (Tsenkova, 2007) could be deployed to get more or different information and to measure the watery samples direct without any sample preparation such as drying.

Western and traditional Chinese medical practices have totally different philosophies and it is a big challenge to apply modern technologies for quality control to very complex products which have been used for centuries. The system of TCM has a characteristic of a complex mixture of hundreds of different chemical substances within the herb with the active principles being partly unknown. Currently in the best case only a few markers of active compounds are used for evaluation of the quality and authenticity. Therefore there is the demand for fingerprint analysis and following this, vibrational spectroscopy could play an important role regarding this approach (Liang *et al.*, 2004; Hai-long *et al.*, 2011).

12.4 Summary

This short article demonstrates that NIR is a promising analytical technique for quality control of raw materials, intermediates and final products in the phyto-pharmaceutical production process of traditional Chinese herbal medicines. Due to its many advantages listed below, NIR in combination with multivariate data analysis has a high potential to become a widely used tool for routine analysis in the production process of traditional Chinese herbal medicine products, especially regarding the implementation of process analytical technology (PAT):

- non-invasive;
- simultaneous determination of physical and chemical properties;
- short analysis time;
- high throughput analysis;
- easy measurement; and
- no/almost no sample preparation necessary.

Together with the rapid development of new chemometric algorithms, faster data processing and enhanced instrumentation, all these advantages would allow NIRS to be deployed for a growing number of new applications for quantitative and qualitative analysis.

Acknowledgments

The authors want to thank Eurasia-Pacific Uninet (EPU) (Salzburg, Austria), the Ministry for Science and Research and the Ministry for Health, Family and Youth (Vienna, Austria) (Novel Analytical Tools for Quality Control in Traditional Chinese Medicine, Project No. 80855), the Leopold-Franzens University, Innsbruck (Nachwuchsförderung) for financial support.

References

Chan, C.O., Chu, C.C., Mok, D.K.W. and Chau, F.T. (2007) Analysis of berberine and total alkaloid content in Cortex Phellodendri by near infrared spectroscopy (NIRS) compared with high-performance liquid chromatography coupled with ultra-visible spectrometric detection. *Anal. Chim. Acta* **592**, 121–131.

Chen, Y., Xie, M.Y., Yan, Y., Zhu, S.B., Nie, S.P., Li, C., Wang, Y.X. and Gong, X.F. (2008) Discrimination of *Ganoderma lucidum* according to geographical origin with near infrared diffuse reflectance spectroscopy and pattern recognition techniques. *Anal. Chim. Acta* **618**, 121–130.

De Smet, P.A. (2005) Herbal medicine in Europe — relaxing regulatory standards. *N. Engl. J. Med.* **352**, 1176–1178.

Fu, H.Y., Huan, S.Y., Xu, L., Jiang, J.H., Wu, H.L., Shen, G.L. and Yu, R.Q. (2009) Construction of an efficacious model for a nondestructive identification of traditional Chinese medicines Liuwei Dihuang pills from different manufacturers using near-infrared spectroscopy and moving window partial least-squares discriminant analysis. *Anal. Sci.* **25**, 1143–1148.

Guo, P., Huang, Q., Zhang, P., Bittner, L., Pezzei, C., Pallua, J. Schonbichler, S., Huck-Pezzei, A., Bonn, K. and Huck, W. (2011) Application of near-infrared spectroscopy (NIRS) as a tool for quality control in traditional chinese medicine (TCM). *Curr. Bioact. Compd.* **7**, 75–84.

Han, B., Chen, N. and Yao, Y. (2009) Discrimination of *radix pseudostellariae* according to geographical origin by FT-NIR spectroscopy and supervised pattern recognition. *Pharmacognos. Mag.* **5**, 279–286.

Huck, C., Maurer, R., Popp, M., Basener, N. and Bonn, G. (1999) Quantitative fourier transform near infrared reflectance spectroscopy (NIRS) compared to high performance liquid chromatography (HPLC) of a flavone in Primulae veris Flos extracts. *Pharm. Pharmacol. Lett.* **9**, 26–29.

Huck, C.W., Abel, G., Popp, M. and Bonn, G.K. (2006) Comparative analysis of naphthodianthrone and phloroglucine derivatives in St. John's Wort extracts by near infrared spectroscopy, high-performance liquid chromatography and capillary electrophoresis. *Anal. Chim. Acta* **580**, 223–230.

Jiang, Y., David, B., Tu, P. and Barbin, Y. (2010) Recent analytical approaches in quality control of traditional Chinese medicines — a review. *Anal. Chim. Acta* **657**, 9–18.

Lai, Y., Ni, Y. and Kokot, S. (2011) Discrimination of Rhizoma corydalis from two sources by near-infrared spectroscopy supported by the wavelet transform and least-squares support vector machine methods. *Vib. Spectrosc.* **56**, 154–160.

Lau, C.C., Chan, C.O., Chau, F.T. and Mok, D.K.W. (2009) Rapid analysis of *Radix puerariae* by near-infrared spectroscopy. *J. Chromatogr. A* **1216**, 2130–2135.

Li, W., Xing, L., Fang, L., Wang, J. and Qu, H. (2010) Application of near infrared spectroscopy for rapid analysis of intermediates of Tanreqing injection. *J. Pharm. Biomed. Anal.* **53**, 350–358.

Liang, Y.Z., Xie, P. and Chan, K. (2004) Quality control of herbal medicines. *J. Chromatogr. B* **812**, 53–70.

Lu, J., Xiang, B., Liu, H., Xiang, S., Xie, S. and Deng, H. (2008) Application of two-dimensional near-infrared correlation spectroscopy to the discrimination of Chinese herbal medicine of different geographic regions. *Spectrochim. Acta A* **69**, 580–586.

Nanlin, Y., Yiyu, C. and Haibin, Q. (2003) Quantitative determination of mannitol in *Cordyceps sinensis* using near infrared spectroscopy and artificial neural networks. *Chin. J. Anal. Chem.* **31**, 664–668.

Robinson, M.M. and Zhang, X. (2011) Traditional medicines: global situation, issues and challenges. In: *The World Medicines Situation 2011*. World Health Organization.

Rosa, S.S., Barata, P.A., Martins, J.M. and Menezes, J.C. (2008) Near-infrared reflectance spectroscopy as a process analytical technology tool in Ginkgo biloba extract qualification. *J. Pharm. Biomed. Anal.* **47**, 320–327.

Tang, Y., Zhang, Z. and Fan, G. (2004) Identification of official rhubarb samples based on NIR spectra and neural networks. *Spectrosc. Spec. Anal.* **24**, 1348–1351.

Tsenkova, R. (2007) AquaPhotomics: Water absorbance pattern as a biological marker for disease diagnosis and disease understanding. *J. Near Infrared Spectrosc.* **18**, 14.

Wang, L., Lee, F.S.C. and Wang, X. (2007) Near-infrared spectroscopy for classification of licorice (*Glycyrrhizia uralensis* Fisch) and prediction of the glycyrrhizic acid (GA) content. *LWT-Food Sci. Technol.* **40**, 83–88.

Woo, Y., Cho, C., Kim, H., Yang, J. and Seong, K. (2002) Classification of cultivation area of ginseng by near infrared spectroscopy and ICP-AES. *Microchem. J.* **73**, 299–306.

Wu, Y.W., Sun, S.Q., Zhou, Q. and Leung, H.W. (2008) Fourier transform mid-infrared (MIR) and near-infrared (NIR) spectroscopy for rapid quality assessment of Chinese medicine preparation Honghua Oil. *J. Pharm. Biomed. Anal.* **46**, 498–504.

Wu, Y., Zheng, Y., Li, Q., Iqbal, J., Zhang, L., Zhang, W. and Du, Y. (2011) Study on difference between epidermis; phloem and xylem of *Radix ginseng* with near-infrared and infrared spectroscopy coupled with principal component analysis. *Vib. Spectrosc.* **55**(2), 201–206.

Xiang, L., Fan, G., Li, J., Kang, H., Yan, Y., Zheng, J. and Guo, D. (2002) The application of an artificial neural network in the identification of medicinal rhubarbs by near infrared spectroscopy. *Phytochem. Anal.* **13**, 272–276.

Yuan, H.-L, Zhang, T.T. and Xiao, X.-H. (2011) Quality control pproaches for Chinese herbal medicines. *Chin. Herb. Med.* **3**, 17–22.

Zhao, L., Zhang, L., Li, J. and Yang, F. (2008) Application of wavelet packet entropy and Fisher classifier to the identification of medicinal rhubarbs with near-infrared spectrum. *Spectrosc. Spectral Anal.* **28**, 817–820.

Index